THE RESPIRATORY FUNCTION
OF THE BLOOD

PART I
LESSONS FROM HIGH ALTITUDES

THE RESPIRATORY FUNCTION OF THE BLOOD

PART I
LESSONS FROM HIGH ALTITUDES

by

JOSEPH BARCROFT
Fellow of King's College, Cambridge

CAMBRIDGE
AT THE UNIVERSITY PRESS
1925

CAMBRIDGE
UNIVERSITY PRESS

University Printing House, Cambridge CB2 8BS, United Kingdom

Published in the United States of America by Cambridge University Press, New York

Cambridge University Press is part of the University of Cambridge.

It furthers the University's mission by disseminating knowledge in the pursuit of education, learning and research at the highest international levels of excellence.

www.cambridge.org
Information on this title: www.cambridge.org/9781107415843

© Cambridge University Press 1925

First published 1925
First paperback edition 2014

A catalogue record for this publication is available from the British Library

ISBN 978-1-107-41584-3 Paperback

TO THE MEMBERS OF MY
PARTY IN SOUTH AMERICA

C. A. BINGER
A. V. BOCK
J. H. DOGGART
H. S. FORBES
G. A. HARROP
J. C. MEAKINS
A. C. REDFIELD

PREFACE

TO THE FIRST EDITION OF
THE RESPIRATORY FUNCTION OF THE BLOOD

At one time, which seems too long ago, most of my leisure was spent in boats. In them I learned what little I know of research, not of technique or of physiology, but of the qualities essential to those who would venture beyond the visible horizon.

The story of my physiological "ventures" will be found in the following pages. Sometimes I have sailed single handed, sometimes I have been one of a crew, sometimes I have sent the ship's boat on some expedition without me. Any merit which attaches to my narrative lies in the fact that it is in some sense at first hand. I have refrained from discussing subjects which I have not actually touched, but which might fittingly have been included in a modern account of the blood as a vehicle for oxygen. Such are the relation of narcosis to oxygen-want and the properties of intracellular oxidative enzymes. The omission of these and other important subjects has made the choice of a title somewhat difficult. I should like to have called the book, what it frankly is—a log; did not such a title involve an air of flippancy quite out of place in the description of the serious work of a man's life. I have therefore chosen a less exact, though more comprehensive title.

After all, the pleasantest memories of a cruise are those of the men with whom one has sailed. The debt which I owe to my colleagues, whether older or younger than myself, will be evident enough to any reader of the book. It leaves me well-nigh bankrupt—a condition well known to most sailors. But I owe another large debt of gratitude to those who, as teachers, showed me the fascination of physiology, to Dr Kimmins *, and especially to

* Formerly science master at the Leys School, now Chief Inspector of the Educational Department of the London County Council.

Dr Anderson *. At a later stage I learned much from Dr Gaskell, Professor Langley and Dr Haldane.

There are occasions on which every sailor of the deep sea has to ship a pilot. Mr A. V. Hill has brought me into those harbours which are best approached through the, to me, unknown channels of mathematics.

* Formerly supervisor in physiology to King's College, now Master of Gonville and Caius College.

J. B.

CAMBRIDGE,
December, 1913.

PREFACE
TO
LESSONS FROM HIGH ALTITUDES

THE rapid advance of knowledge rendered impossible the task of revising *The Respiratory Function of the Blood* for a second edition. The book was in three parts with an Appendix on technique: there is now more than enough known about the subject-matter of each part to justify a book on that alone. I have therefore determined to break up the volume into a *series* of manageable units, originally intended to correspond more or less to the "Parts" of the original work. The first volume of this series is now presented.

I have to thank the Royal Society for permission to reproduce Figs. 10, 11, 12, 13, 14, 15, 17, 18, 25, 26, 29, 30, 37, 41, 42, 44, 45, 46, 48 and 50; *Physiological Review*, Figs. 31, 32, 33, 34; *Journal of Physiology*, Figs. 23, 24; *R.A.M.C. Journal*, Figs. 22, 39, 40; *Quarterly Journal of Medicine*, Figs. 20 and 38; the Medical Research Council, Figs. 35 and 36; the Peruvian Corporation, Fig. 3; *Nature*, Fig. 16, and my friends Dr Douglas for the plates of Figs. 1, 7, 8 and 9, Professor Durig for that of Fig. 5, and Professor Aggazzotti for those of Figs. 4 and 6.

J. B.

CAMBRIDGE,
September, 1925.

CONTENTS

CHAPTER I

MOUNTAIN SICKNESS AND ITS CAUSE

WITHIN the span of life of the middle aged a wonderful change has come over our knowledge of the causation of disease. Indeed to say that nothing was known about the matter in the early seventies of last century is not very far from the fact.

Since that date the whole science of bacteriology has arisen, the micro-organisms which are responsible for innumerable complaints have been isolated. By analogy we argue that certain other diseases are communicated by similar agents, and in some of the most remarkable researches of our time the insects by which these micro-organisms are disseminated have been sought out. Nowadays there is before us a complete panorama of the ætiology of epidemics, no single component of which was vouchsafed to those who died about the time of my own birth. I well remember being rebuked for sleeping with the window open not on the ground that by such action I courted the mosquito, but for such reasons as that "the night air was injurious" or that "to sleep in a draught was certain to give me a cold which might lead to inflammation of the lungs or even consumption."

In those days therefore any disorder which had a definite cause loomed large for the student of medical science—among such was mountain sickness. Most persons as they approached the snow line in the Alps were inclined to vomit. Sometimes the inclination overcame them. In other cases severe headache ensued and so forth, but the cause seemed clear, it was the ascent into the rarer levels of the atmosphere.

Indeed according to Longstaff[1] (1), these scientific investigators were the fathers of mountaineering. "During the latter part of the eighteenth and the beginning of the nineteenth century, that great period of awakening interest and research into physical science, mountain ascents were encouraged and performed only by scientific men. Such men, practised observers and expecting to be severely affected by what we consider to be only moderate diminutions in atmospheric pressure noted even the smallest abnormal symptoms

[1] Dr Longstaff's paper was published in 1906 when much less was known about anoxæmia than at present. Probably being a doctor, his point of view has shifted, but it represents that of many climbers who are not medical men.

in themselves....On the other hand during the last fifty years mountaineering has become a sport and is practised by a much larger and very different class, although it is true that many men of scientific attainments are to be found in the ranks of modern mountaineers."

Whether or no these early scientists were inclined to exaggerate their symptoms, as Longstaff suggests, their modern brothers will endorse the view that the cause of their complaint was the diminished partial pressure of oxygen in the lung. This view which seemed to be established by the researches of Paul Bert (2) has been challenged seriously on two occasions, once by Dr Longstaff himself, and once by the Italian physiologist Mosso. Longstaff considered[1] that mountain sickness was due to a combination of physical exertion, "want of condition," and poverty of diet. The general trend of his argument may be gleaned from the following quotation. "In support of this view I would mention the ascents of the Peak of Teneriffe (12,200 feet) and of Fujiyama (12,425 feet). These are both easy walks. They are frequently climbed by tourists who have no experience of mountaineering and generally, owing to their geographical position, at the end of a sea voyage. The ascents take two days from the sea-level and have to be done on foot so that there is no rapid change in pressure. Yet on both these mountains reports of mountain sickness, often of a severe type, are of very frequent occurrence. I maintain that there are no sufficient grounds for attributing these cases primarily to insufficient oxygen. If these people were placed in a pneumatic chamber and the pressure reduced to an equivalent extent it is almost certain that they would remain unaffected by so slight a diminution in O_2 supply. But these individuals have performed an enormous physical task, such a task as they have probably never previously attempted and for which they are not in proper training. It would be surprising if great physiological disturbances did not arise under conditions which must produce an extreme degree of fatigue."

Much confusion seems to have arisen from the basing of argument on individual cases, and therefore it is with a good deal of diffidence that I cite my own experiences in criticism of a statement made by so great an authority on mountaineering as Dr Longstaff. It does happen that I have been the witness, and in one case the victim, of experiments which appear to be the obvious "controls" to Dr Longstaff's statement.

[1] In 1906.

Firstly, I have seen the summit of Teneriffe climbed by persons who started only 1500 feet below it, perfectly fresh and in good condition, and secondly, I have lived in "chambers" in diminished partial pressure of oxygen.

About Fujiyama I can say nothing, but about Teneriffe I can testify that our party had avoided all the causes to which Long-staff attributes mountain sickness. They had lived and walked a good deal and been excellently fed at an altitude of 7000 feet for

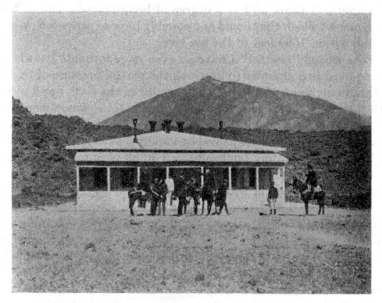

FIG. 1. The summit of Teneriffe as seen from the Cañadas. The white patch just below the summit is pumice above which is sand.

a fortnight, so that they only had 5000 feet to ascend. Of these they climbed all but 1500 feet on mules and even then two slept the night in the hut at 10,800 feet before the crater was climbed. Prof. Zuntz's expedition had not performed any fatiguing feat before their ascent. The actual climbing of the last five 500 can only be described as "an easy walk," in the sense (and that no doubt is what Longstaff means) of being quite devoid of mountaineering difficulties.

Considered in the light of the amount of energy which must be expended per foot of ascent accomplished the climbing is far from easy. The surface of the ground at the summit of the peak consists of sand which lies at the critical angle; as the tourist endeavours to climb, the ground beneath him sinks immediately his weight is placed upon it. For every foot he goes up he comes down nine inches. The party of which Douglas and I formed two members, arrived at the Alta Vista Hut perfectly fresh and in good condition, but the 1500 feet which remained to be climbed, entailed a greater expenditure of energy than is usually required for so trivial an ascent. Of the party of seven one was so mountain sick as to turn back, the rest all reached the summit. I think all felt a degree of breathlessness and at least two a nausea which they could not possibly have experienced on such a climb within 1500 feet of the sea level.

Of the second "control" I have an even more intimate knowledge, having lived in a chamber (4) in which the partial pressure of oxygen was gradually reduced until on the morning of the sixth day I awoke with three of the typical symptoms of mountain sickness, vomiting, intense headache and difficulty of vision. I have recollections of very acute headache accompanied by vomiting as a child, but never in adult life or even in my boyhood can I think of any such attack as occurred in the chamber, there seems to be no reason to regard it as an attack of megrain which "just happened" to occur that day. In the chamber I had lived an easy though normal life, reading, writing, making observations, doing gas analysis, cleaning the chamber, seeing to the air scrubbers, taking exercise on the bicycle ergometer and so forth. Moreover I had been thoroughly well fed— a rather light breakfast, tea, eggs, bread and butter cooked by the attendant and lunch and dinner sent from the College kitchens. There was no cause other than oxygen want to which my sickness could be attributed. It is true, of course, that the partial pressure of oxygen corresponded to about 18,000 feet and therefore a much higher altitude than that of the Peak of Teneriffe but, on the other hand, I had not precipitated matters by the performance of any such exacting feat as the ascent of a sandhill 1500 feet in height. There is every reason to suppose that my friend who was sick on Teneriffe would have been sick doing the same amount of work in a chamber in which the oxygen pressure was that to which he was subjected on the Peak and would not have been sick under similar circumstances in atmospheric air. And this brings me to the undoubted element of truth which runs through the whole of Longstaff's—as it seems to me—vicious argument. Fatigue, of course, is an element in mountain

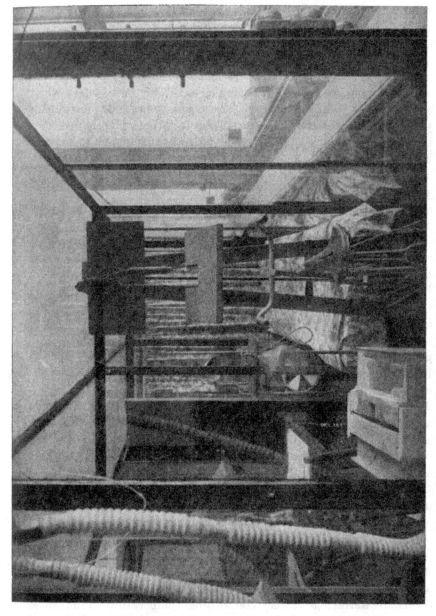

FIG. 2. Glass respiration chamber in the Physiological Laboratory, Cambridge, England.

sickness, for mountain sickness is due to *oxygen want* and oxygen want is the discrepancy between oxygen supply and oxygen demand. It depends upon the balance between the two. The mountain sickness complex may be brought on at almost any given altitude at which the demand of the body for oxygen can be made to exceed the supply to a sufficient degree and for a sufficient time. The vice of Longstaff's argument consists in his presenting as antithetic two factors which are in reality complementary. There could be no more convincing proof that mountain sickness is not due to fatigue than is furnished by the passengers who daily reach altitudes of about 15,000 feet by train. A vivid account (5) has been given by Haldane and his colleagues of the condition of the tourists who were conveyed to the summit of Pike's Peak during the stay there of the party. Even more convincing, if possible, is the exhibition which daily takes place at

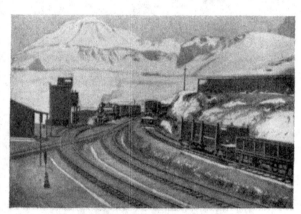

FIG. 3. Ticlio near the summit of the Central Railway of Peru.

Ticlio the highest point of the Central Railway of Peru. It would seem that here the effect of the rare atmosphere is more immediate than at Pike's Peak, for this there may be several reasons. In the first place, the altitude is somewhat higher being just short of 16,000 feet at the highest point (15,885 feet to be exact), in the second place, the train conveys not merely tourists whose object is to ascend the mountain, but all and sundry—men, women and children who are crossing the Andes in the course of their business, and in the third place, the train when on its journey east comes up the whole way from the sea level in less than twelve hours. Unlike ascents on the Alps, the element of cold may be ruled out as constituting a possible cause of the sickness of the passengers who reach Ticlio for the trains are warmed to a very comfortable temperature. It must be admitted that when first I passed over this summit I was occupied in keeping very quiet lest I should be sick myself—an effort which proved to be abortive, for while I was not actually sick in the train, the crisis came two or three hours later when I left the train at an altitude of 12,000 feet. On the occasion of my second crossing I was in a better position to observe my neighbours, looking out at Ticlio I saw the most astonishing spectacle; all along the train from the windows of the carriages occupied by οἱ πολλοί, a row of heads protruded from the windows—the outward and visible sign of a single purpose, that of regurgitation.

Of course there are more subtle factors involved in mountain sickness than diminished pressure of oxygen in the lungs and the degree of muscular exercise which is involved. An instance is the sight of food. I remember having a bad quarter of an hour at the Capanna Margherita on the most accessible summit of Monte Rosa. I had been there twenty hours without any tendency to mountain sickness and I had slept reasonably well, but lunch was almost too much. I struggled through without the nausea turning into anything worse, but I ate little and just sipped at a glass of wine. In the last resort the symptoms of mountain sickness are less due to deficient oxygen supply to the body as a whole, than to deficient oxygen supply to the brain; if therefore the amount of oxygen which is reaching the brain at any moment be only just sufficient, a diversion of blood from the brain to other regions whether the cause be physical or psychological may precipitate mountain sickness.

Another point made by Longstaff has perhaps received too little attention, namely, the factor of cold. He quotes the work of Zuntz, Schumberg and Loewy [6] who found a 40 per cent. increase of oxygen consumption by the human body when at rest on Monte Rosa. At Cerro de Pasco, in Peru, at an altitude of 14,200 feet we recorded no such experience. Out of five cases studied the change in oxygen consumption was as follows [7]:

Meakins's oxygen intake at rest rose 25 per cent.
Harrop's　　　　,,　　　　,,　　,, 15　,,
Binger's　　　　,,　　　　,,　　,, 4　,,
Redfield's　　　　,,　　　　,, fell 2　,,
Barcroft's　　　　,,　　　　,,　　,, 15　,,
Bock's　　　　,,　　　　,,　　,, 12　,,

When I enquire as to what may be the caus of the discrepancy between Zuntz's results and our own my mind g es back to the night which I spent shivering on Monte Rosa and to he contrast between the conditions there and those of the beautifu little cottage where we were housed at Cerro and in which there was a large fire-place and as hot a bath as you please. The mere fact of living at an altitude of 14,000 feet does not send up my oxygen consumption, but in Cambridge by going from my own laboratory to that of the cold storage research department and sitting at 0° till I feel inclined to shiver, I can put up my oxygen consumption by one-sixth and I have seen that of my colleague, E. K. Marshall, rise from 269 to 410 c.c. per minute (66 per cent.) by the same procedure[8]. Cold then, in so far as it raises the oxygen consumption is equivalent to work, and does so by increasing the muscular contraction. To that extent it is a predisposing cause of oxygen want.

The second theory of mountain sickness which has had some vogue is that of Mosso[3] who was impressed by the fact that there was less carbonic acid in the expired air at high altitudes than is normally the case.

Further reference to this theory will be made in the chapter on the hydrogen-ion concentration of the blood. Here it need only be said that, so far as I know, the theory is dead. For me it died when I was on the Peak of Teneriffe when first at the Alta Vista Hut (10,500 feet) without actually vomiting I was a good deal affected by the altitude, Douglas who was with me was quite unaffected. Yet the carbonic acid in my alveolar air was practically normal, in his it was reduced[9].

	CO_2 pressure in England	Alveolar air mm. Alta Vista
Barcroft	40	38
Douglas	39–42	31·9

Douglas was well though acapnic, I was not acapnic yet ailing. Granting one's CO_2 production to be the same at the Alta Vista Hut as normal it follows that the fall in Douglas's CO_2 was due to increased total ventilation, which in my case, unfortunately, did not take place. It may be deduced that because my alveolar CO_2 was six millimetres higher than that of Douglas my alveolar oxygen was seven or eight millimetres lower and this no doubt was the cause of my trouble.

Whilst there can be no doubt that oxygen want is the prime cause of mountain sickness there remain some rather interesting points which have never been quite cleared up, one of these is the persistent statements that as between localities situated at the same altitude mountain sickness is more prevalent at some than at others. In general, for instance, persons are said to be affected at lower altitudes in the Andes than in the Himalayas. Of course it is not a foregone conclusion that at equal altitudes the barometric pressure is the same in Thibet as in Peru, any more than the level of the sea is the same in the Atlantic and in the Pacific. In point of fact the sea level at one end of the Panama Canal is appreciably different from that at the other. I put the question to Sir Napier Shaw who very kindly supplied me with such statistics as there are on the subject. They went to show that there was a slight difference in the mean barometric readings at say 15,000 feet as between the Andes and the Himalayas, but as the barometer is on the whole higher in the Andes the trifling difference of atmospheric pressure renders alleged proneness to mountain sickness in the Cordilleras of Peru the more remarkable.

The late Dr Kellas in an unpublished manuscript, from which the secretary of the Alpine Club has kindly given me permission to quote, makes the following remarks on this subject: "Zuntz has also pointed out that Mountain Sickness seems to vary greatly in incidence with locality. He observes that it is met with at 3000 metres in the Alps and Caucasus, at 4000 metres in the Andes and at 5000 metres in the Himalayas.

"This statement would be very difficult of explanation if true, since the composition of the atmosphere is practically uniform, except with regard to relative humidity, but it can only be considered a vague generalisation, expressing the chances of acclimatisation. As indicated later, if untrained individuals can rapidly alter their altitude mountain sickness may be produced, but if the alteration is slow acclimatisation prevents incidence. Hooker[10] for example states that they never suffered when riding at 18,000 feet in the Himalaya (where the traveller by road generally takes at least a week to reach 15,000 feet) but he suffered when climbing on foot.

"More important because more difficult of explanation is the statement, that mountain sickness varies within certain narrow areas. Two general statements have been made in this connection.

"(1) It has been repeatedly affirmed by travellers and natives of the Himalaya and Andes that passes of about the same height in the same region differ greatly as regards incidence of mountain sickness. For example v. Tschudi[11] states that it is incident with great severity in some districts in Peru, whilst in others of higher altitude it is scarcely perceptible.

"(2) It has also been generally assumed that one is more liable to be attacked when climbing in gullies and on snow, than on open ridges and rock.

"Many quotations might be given regarding this latter statement. De Saussure (12) in describing the early unsuccessful attempts on Mont Blanc says that in 1783 two chamois hunters ascended by a series of rock arêtes to within 2500 feet of the summit, and that 'the air on those slopes was so easy and light that there was no fear of that kind of suffocation felt in the valley of snow, which extended from the mountain of La Coté at a lower elevation, which had defeated another attempt during the same year.

"In 1831 Boussingault (13) wrote in connection with his attempt on Chimborazo "A hauteur égale, je crois avoir remarqué, que l'on respire plus difficilement sur la neige, que lorsque l'on se trouve sur un rocher." Conway in connection with the ascent of Pioneer Peak remarks that they felt much worse on snow than on the arête, in fact they had difficulty in restraining themselves from taking to the cornice[1].

"Thomas on the contrary found climbing on rocks more difficult than on snow, suggesting that the heated rocks caused rarefaction of the air, agreeing with Zurbiggen, a guide of quite exceptional ability and experience, who told Professor Mosso that he suffered more on bare mountains than on snow or ice.

"Probably all these vague statements are capable of simple explanation. It seems unnecessary to invoke ionisation of the air due to radio-activity of the minerals present in certain mountain regions, a theory due to Zuntz. Intense electrical disturbances which would produce ionisation seem to have little effect on the incidence of mountain sickness, but Mosso cites examples of an apparent influence, perhaps psychic in origin.

"The true explanation of the above contradictory statements regarding incidence of mountain sickness is probably much simpler, but may depend upon several factors, all of which would require to be considered in any particular case:

"(a) Nature of the ground, e.g. whether snow or rock, and whether easy or difficult.

"(b) Presence or absence of wind.

[1] Major R. W. G. Hingston, I.M.S., medical officer to the 1924 Everest expedition draws especial attention to this point, under the heading of Glacier Lassitude. The discomfort felt on snow and glaciers especially when in enclosed places is attributed to a high degree of saturation of the atmosphere with aqueous vapour. [*Proceedings of the Royal Geographical Society*, 10 Nov. 1924.]

"(c) Possible deficiency or alteration of diet as compared with normal.

"(d) Weather."

In considering the explanation of the fact that at a given altitude mountain sickness seems to be more in evidence at some places than in others it is necessary to get back to the fundamental point and to remember two things: firstly, that mountain sickness is due to oxygen want, and secondly, that it is due to oxygen want on the part of the medulla. Thus under any particular circumstances we have got to consider:

(1) Are the circumstances such as to increase the oxygen want of the system generally?

(2) If so is such a general condition of oxygen want likely to fall on the medulla?

(3) Are there any special reasons why it should fall especially on the medulla?

With regard to the first question, if the oxygen pressure in the lungs is so low that the arterial blood is less than 90 per cent. saturated with oxygen, any untoward effort tends to reduce the oxygen pressure in it still further, therefore, unless there is some compensation such as an increase of blood supply in the brain, the supply of oxygen to the medulla will fall off. That is the answer to the second question. Therefore if it is a greater effort to lift the legs through deep snow than to walk along rock, one might expect a correspondingly greater tendency to mountain sickness. Again, if there were any conditions which would tend to divert blood from the brain to other parts of the body, the medulla would suffer correspondingly.

At present our knowledge of the blood supply to the brain is extremely limited, a further reference will be made to the matter when we discuss the subject of acclimatisation. In the meantime we may leave the matter with the statement that there appear to be abundant possibilities of blood supply to the brain being altered by varying circumstances at a critical altitude and therefore of the effects of oxygen want being precipitated or warded off.

Different persons experience mountain sickness at very varying altitudes. Let us leave out of account the "subjective factor"—that mystery which makes all experiments on man so difficult and which makes experiments in biological science so different from those in chemistry and physics. In chemistry the factors are all known and if the factors with which one is dealing have been mastered the reagents can be made to behave in precisely the same manner time after time. Not so with man—"What is one man's food is another man's poison." The dose which will produce profound symptoms in one person will pass as harmless to his neighbour. When I allude to this as a mystery I mean only that our ignorance is profound. In the case of mountain sickness we may however consider one specific difference, or possible difference between different persons, namely, the difference in the permeability of the lung to oxygen. I will leave for the present the general permeability of the lung and consider only the fact that certain portions of the lung may function but indifferently. Suppose, for instance, that a certain part of the lung becomes less elastic than the rest (which it might do as the result of some old inflammatory or other trouble) what would be the result? At each inspiration the air would not be changed so thoroughly in the inelastic portion as in the remainder of the lung. Under ordinary circumstances, the deficiency in ventilation might not matter because, though the oxygen pressure in this part of the lung is less than else-where, it might yet be sufficient to aerate the blood which traverses its wall. Thus if the general oxygen pressure in the lung were 110 mm. and that in the poorly ventilated portion were 85 mm., there would only be a trifling difference in the bloods leaving the two portions, and the mixed blood would be practically unaltered in composition. If, however, the oxygen pressure in the well ventilated portion was 50 mm. and that in the poorly ventilated portion was 25 mm. of mercury, the difference in saturation of the bloods from the two portions would be very great. If then the ill-ventilated portion con-stituted an appreciable fraction of the whole lung, the general arterial blood would be sensibly more deficient in oxygen than that of a normal person. Hence the possessor of such a lung, other things being equal, would suffer from mountain sickness at a much lower altitude. Great stress has been laid in recent years on the unequal ventilation of various lung areas, especially by Haldane. Whether such a phenomenon is a noteworthy factor in the respiration of normal lungs, I do not propose here to discuss; but I would emphasise the fact that even in a lung in which the ventilation is at normal levels sufficiently uniform for practical purpose, the deficiency in ventilation caused by some old fibrosis may be calamitous at high altitudes.

Let us pass to the consideration of the symptoms of mountain sickness, to some statement of what the term embraces and to its claim to be a complaint which manifests itself in such various ways to rank as a "clinical entity." Dr A. C. Redfield, in a manuscript which he kindly sent me, has treated these questions so admirably that I cannot do better than give his description:

"In the Andes the disability which most men suffer on coming into the rarified air is termed 'seroche.' So definite is its symptomatology, so general is its occurrence in these not unpopulous regions, that it deserves some attention as a clinical entity. Its severity is sufficient to give it, in connection with the mining industry, a certain economic importance. While a few men were met who had never felt it and many who had suffered but mildly, a very large number are so greatly affected as to be completely incapacitated for several days. In at least one authentic instance the 'seroche' of a normal healthy person has been terminated by death.

"Each case is an individual story and up to the present no one has been able to predict who will and who will not be affected. A description of cases of two degrees of severity will serve to picture the chief features of the disorder.

"Making the ascent by train, one lightly touched by 'seroche' experiences his first symptoms at an altitude of 10,000 feet or more. Subjectively lassitude, then headache, usually frontal, growing in severity, and perhaps nausea are felt. One feels cold, particularly in the extremities, the pulse quickens, respiration becomes deeper and more frequent, the face is pallid, lips and nails are cyanotic. On descending from the summit to Oroya at 12,000 feet, though a marked improvement is felt one finds himself reduced to a helpless condition of weakness which renders the least muscular effort irksome and productive of shortness of breath, dizziness, and palpitation. The night's sleep is restless and on waking one feels much as he does on venturing on to his feet after recovering from an acute infection. In two or three days, one's strength returns, the colour improves somewhat and all but the more severe forms of exertion may be undertaken without distress. The majority are less fortunate than this. During the ascent the symptoms are qualitatively the same, but frequently more severe, and nausea gives way to vomiting. The night's sleep fails to bring relief; severe headache, gastro-intestinal instability, and weakness continue for several days; the body temperature may be supranormal (102° F. by rectum), and at times one is aware of palpitation. Cyanosis is marked. After three or four days in bed, relief comes and in a week normal activity may be resumed."

The following more detailed account, especially of the symptoms, of our own party in Peru is taken from our report in the *Philosophical Transactions of the Royal Society* (7):

The untoward symptoms which the members of the party experienced at Oroya (12,000 feet) and Cerro de Pasco (14,300 feet) may best be considered under two heads. First, those acute symptoms which came on the first or second day after arrival, and secondly those symptoms which persisted in perhaps lessening degree throughout the sojourn at high altitudes. To the first group of symptoms the name of "seroche" is generally applied. These are sufficiently outspoken, though variable in their manifestation, to constitute what might be called a "clinical entity." Of the eight members of the party four had "seroche" in sufficiently severe degree to force them to go to bed from one to four days. Rest in bed was as imperative to their feeling of well-being as it would be to a patient in the first few days of an acute infection. The remaining four all had symptoms but not severe enough to disable them. After the acute "seroche" subsided all members of the group were able to put in a good day's work of nine to ten hours' duration in the laboratory. The table of symptoms refers to those felt at any time during the period of exposure to low atmospheric pressures.

A few excerpts taken from diaries of members of the party will describe the onset and course of symptoms perhaps better than any attempt at a more general description of the illness.

I. *Example of a mild case.*

Dec. 19. Rail road.

> Tamborague 9826 ft. Pulse 64.
> San Mateo 10,534 ft. Pulse 74. Respirations more marked. Thoracic in type. Loosened my waistcoat and belt. Felt distinctly inclined to sit still.
> Rio Blanco 11,430 ft. Pulse 78. Felt a bit light-headed and cold in my feet.
> Casapalca 13,606 ft. I began to feel really badly with a good vigorous headache and a slight feeling of nausea. Feet and hands cold—chilly sensations.
> Yauli 13,420 ft. Headache practically gone.
> Oroya 12,178 ft. Pretty winded in lifting baggage out of car window.

Dec. 20. I feel exactly as one does on the first day out after a week of tonsilitis or grippe. Unsteady on my pins. Walked about very slowly perhaps ⅛ of a mile—my legs ached as if I had walked 30 miles.

Dec. 23. Spent a.m. straightening up car and walked back to house. Climbed up hill 100 ft. without undue blowing. Ran part of the way from house to hospital without getting winded.

II. *Example of a more severe case of short duration.*

Dec. 23–24. Arrived Cerro de Pasco (14,300 ft.) about 10 p.m. Felt very well probably rather euphoric. During night severe headache behind the eyes and in occipital region. In a.m. rather deaf and my vision was very dim. I had photophobia and felt very irritable. No appetite. Could not sleep. Muscular pain in back and thighs. Rectal temperature 100° F.

Dec. 26. Attack cleared up and I felt in normal condition again.

III.

Dec. 21. Casapalca (13,606 ft.).

3.10 p.m. Drowsiness, headache, malaise, slight cyanosis.

3.20 ,, Slightly deaf and can't see very well.

4.00 ,, Ticlio (15,885 ft.). Severe frontal and parietal headache. Feel rotten —lying down. Cyanosed—dim vision—nausea. Difficult to reply to questions.

4.20 ,, Vomited.

4.30 ,, Vomited again—grey cyanosis.

Oroya (12,178 ft.). Lying back with eyes closed.

5.30 ,, Able to walk from train to auto. Very dizzy, splitting headache. Taken directly to hospital—put to bed.

Dec. 21–24. In bed with severe headache which prevented sleep. No nausea or vomiting after first night. Weakness. Felt as if I'd been hit with a brick.

Dec. 25. Out of bed. Short of breath. No headache.

IV.

Dec. 19. After headache, shortness of breath and sense of lassitude of gradually increasing severity—the following notes:

R.R. Ticlio. I had only one desire and that was to be horizontal in a warm bed.

Oroya (12,178 ft.). It was about all I could do to handle my big bag. I was winded—splitting headache—teeth chattered. Slightest motion caused my head to ache violently. My face was flushed and lips a dull lavender. Fingernails cyanotic about the base and white at the tips. Hands and feet cold.

Went to bed about midnight. While undressing had a pretty severe chill. Head ached furiously—retrobulbar and occipital. Felt alternately hot and cold. Temporal arteries throbbing. Heart palpitated and felt short of breath. Respirations 24. Pulse 92. Temperature by rectum 102·6° F. Felt as if in the prodromal stage of an acute infectious disease.

Dec. 20 (a.m.). Physical examination negative except for cyanosis, fever and rapid pulse. Lungs clear.

Dec. 21. Temperature normal. General improvement. Headache persists the less.

Dec. 22. Out of bed. Feel weak. Headache still present. Even slow walking produces dyspnœa.

Dec. 23. Cerro de Pasco (14,300 ft.). No ill effect from added altitude.

Dec. 24. Awoke with very severe headache. Stayed in bed till noon. Danced two dances at Xmas Eve Party with slight puffing. No further acute symptoms.

These notes give a fairly representative description of "seroche" as experienced by members of the expedition. More severe types of longer duration and indeed sudden death are described by some—but we have confined our account to what we ourselves have observed.

After the acute symptoms of "seroche" had subsided the effects of the high altitude were manifest in a variety of ways in different individuals. Cyanosis was constantly present in all the members of the party to a greater or less extent. The degree by casual observation was not necessarily indicative of the degree of arterial oxygen saturation. Those individuals who normally had a more or less florid complexion appeared more cyanosed than did those whose appearance was paler. The contrast between the natives and Europeans in this regard was most striking. Practically all the healthy natives were of a "plum colour" in those anatomical areas where arterial blood lends colour to the skin. This was particularly evident in the children. In those native adults where this was not conspicuous it was evident that they were probably suffering from some organic disease, such as miner's phthisis, tuberculosis, etc., or were chronic habitués of cocaine.

We were fortunate to have the opportunity of observing the effect of the altitude upon one of the Anglo-Saxon engineers who has been resident in Cerro de Pasco for some years. He was a man of very powerful physique who was in no manner troubled by the altitude. His cyanosis was of an extreme type but it was also noted that his skin capillaries were particularly prominent and presented the appearance of being extremely well filled. His blood examination showed the red cells to number 6,800,000 and the hæmoglobin to be 128 per cent. He accompanied us to sea-level, where the alteration in his appearance was most remarkable. Instead of being of a deep "plum colour" his complexion was a brilliant red as if he had recently become intensely sunburnt. The change in his appearance was duplicated by certain of our party but he afforded an example which all could observe without prejudice.

The general well-being of the party differed considerably in degree as time passed. It seemed to bear no relation to the severity of the initial symptoms. This probably was to be expected, as those who had suffered from acute "seroche" had had their lesson, and deported themselves in combined work and play more circumspectly than did those who had escaped. The latter, as time passed, showed a distinct slackening of their energy. The desire was unimpaired but the capacity was distinctly lessened. This was particularly evident in so far as prolonged physical exertion was concerned. Not that their capacity was diminished below their fellows but they were comparatively less capable of exertion as time progressed and in consequence they required more rest and were approaching the more sensible attitude of their associates who had been early less fortunate.

In all members of the expedition the effect on the mental processes was insidious but eventually quite apparent. Although short and precise exercises did not exhibit any pronounced change in the nervous and reflex capacity of the members of the party, prolonged concentration gave evidence of lowered control. Whereas at sea-level certain members of the party would use a Haldane gas-analysis apparatus or other similar technique for days on end without a mistake, rarely a day passed at Cerro de Pasco without one or more having to take the apparatus apart and clean it, through some stupid mistake of manipulation.

In the matter of arithmetic similar mistakes were evident. It was not so much that gross errors were made as that frequently simple sums had to be gone over repeatedly before the worker was satisfied as to the accuracy. Like conditions were observed when the slide-rule and logarithms were used.

Although the party worked for long hours on end in the laboratory —it being the custom for certain members to have their lunch and tea there daily—the amount of work accomplished in a day was sometimes disappointing. This was undoubtedly due to the conspicuous mental and physical fatigue which gradually developed as the day wore on, with the inevitable slowness and clumsiness which ensued. This effect of prolonged and steady work was not only confined to the members of the party. Men who had lived at Cerro de Pasco for years without any symptoms of acute "seroche" informed us that the best work in the end was obtained by short periods of work with long rests between. This was particularly the case in those whose occupation was mental—accountants, draftsmen, etc.

It has been stated that life at high altitudes is conducive to irascibility of temper. As far as the present party was concerned this was not evident. On no occasion was any petulance or unreasonableness exhibited by members of the party one to another. On the other hand impatience at one's own mistakes was commonly manifest and usually produced a considerable amount of amusement amongst the rest of the party.

The other symptoms which developed during our stay at Cerro de Pasco were confined to our physical well-being. The appetite was often capricious and irregular. At times it was almost voracious and at others the mere mention of food was distasteful. Sleep was almost uniformly disturbed and not of long duration. Those who were accustomed to 8 to 10 hours' sleep would usually find it impossible to sleep more than 6 to 8 hours. At intervals however certain members of the party who usually slept the least would sleep for 12 to 14 hours on end. One of the most notable features due to the residence at high altitudes was loss of weight. This occurred in all members of the party but more in some than in others. The greatest loss of weight was a decline from 155 pounds to 131 pounds in 27 days. This amount was quickly regained when the individual returned to sea-level. We were informed by those who had lived at high altitudes for some years that an initial loss of weight was almost universal but that a certain amount was subsequently regained although the former sea-level weight was seldom reached.

One party in Peru were extremely fortunate in having the assistance of Dr Crane the principal medical officer of the Cerro de Pasco Copper Corporation. This powerful American Mining Company controls most things in the part of the world in which we were and they were most kind in placing their whole organisation at our disposal. Though it was not definitely put into words, I gathered that there was one reservation, namely, that before welcoming us at the higher altitudes as their guests they were going to assure themselves that our health was such as would not suffer by our residence "on the hill" (as the phrase there goes). My impression is that some fatality, or may be some fiasco, which they did not wish to have repeated, had occurred previously, but whether this was so or not their action was welcomed by us as the truest hospitality. So it happened to each of us when we arrived at Oroya, that we were very kindly but quite firmly dealt with, and each was put to bed in the beautifully equipped little hospital under Dr Crane's supervision and kept there till he was satisfied that the "seroche" had passed off. This might be a night, two nights or longer. How well do I remember being carried on a stretcher from the house of Mr Collie the Head Engineer of the Company—a most delightful person—to the hospital adjacent, and reflecting on the singularity of experiencing for the first time in my life that highest refinement of civilised life, up-to-date hospital treatment, 6000 miles from home, 12,000 feet up in the air and in a region

	C.N.S. symptoms	Cardiac symptoms	Peripheral circulatory symptoms	Respiratory symptoms	Gastro-intestinal symptoms
BARCROFT	Headache+ Lassitude+ Fatigue++ Sleeplessness+	Precordial pain+	Cold extremities+ Cyanosis+	Shortness of breath on exertion+	Nausea+ Vomiting+ Anorexia+
MEAKINS	Restlessness Fatigue+ Bad dreams	Precordial pain+ Palpitation+	Cold extremities+ Throbbing+ Cyanosis+	Shortness of breath+ Periodic breathing+ Sighing+	
DOGGART	Sleeplessness+	—	Cyanosis+	Shortness of breath+ Periodic breathing+ Sighing+	
BINGER	Headache++ Lassitude+ Fatigue+ Sleeplessness+	Precordial pain+ Palpitation+	Chill+ Cold extremities+ Cyanosis+	Shortness of breath on exertion+ Sighing+	Nausea+
BOCK	Headache+++ Sleeplessness+ Visual and auditory impairment+ Lassitude+ Fatigue+	—	Throbbing pulses Feeling of heat and sweating+ Pallor+ Cyanosis++	Shortness of breath++ Sighing++	Nausea+ Vomiting++ Abdominal pain+ Anorexia+
FORBES	Headache+ Vertigo+ Visual disturbance+ Fatigue+ Lassitude Sleeplessness+	Precordial pain+ Palpitation+	Chilly sensations+ Cold extremities+ Cyanosis+ Epistaxis+	Shortness of breath+ Irregular breathing+ Sighing+	Nausea+
HARROP	Headache+++ Visual disturbance+ Auditory disturbance+ Lassitude+ Depression+ Fatigue+ Sleeplessness+	Sinus arrhythmia	Cyanosis Throbbing arteries+	Shortness of breath+ Periodic breathing+ Orthopnœa+ Sighing+	Anorexia
REDFIELD	Headache+ Lassitude+ Fatigue++ Restless sleep	Palpitation+	Cold feet+ Cyanosis+	Shortness of breath+ Periodic breathing+ Sighing	Nausea+

in which a continuous prospect of rock was broken only by the houses of the miners and the streams which form the head-waters of the Amazon.

Dr Crane then, than whom no one has better opportunities of judging of the symptoms and nature of mountain sickness, went over each of our cases and we are indebted to him for many of the details in the above table (p. 19).

BIBLIOGRAPHY

(1) LONGSTAFF. *Mountain Sickness and its Probable Causes.* London, 1906.

(2) PAUL BERT. *La pression barométrique.* 1878.

(3) MOSSO. *Life in the High Alps.*

(4) BARCROFT; COOKE, HARTRIDGE, PARSONS AND PARSONS. *Journ. Physiol.* LIII. 450. 1920.

(5) DOUGLAS, HALDANE, HENDERSON AND SCHNEIDER. *Phil. Trans. Roy. Soc.* B. CCIII. 185. 1912.

(6) ZUNTZ AND SCHUMBERG, ALSO BY LOEWY. Numerous papers chiefly in *Pflüger's Archiv,* 1895–1902.

(7) BARCROFT; BINGER, BOCK, DOGGART, FORBES, HARROP, MEAKINS AND REDFIELD. *Phil. Trans. Roy. Soc.* B. CCXI. 351. 1923.

(8) BARCROFT AND MARSHALL. *Journ. Physiol.* LVIII. 145. 1923.

(9) BARCROFT. *Journ. Physiol.* XLII. 63. 1911.

(10) HOOKER. *Himalayan Journals.*

(11) TSCHUDI. (Peru.) *Reiseskizzen,* 1838–42.

(12) DE SAUSSURE. *Voyages dans les Alpes.*

(13) BOUSSINGAULT AND HALL. *Gay Lussac's Ann. de Chimie et de Physique.*

CHAPTER II

SOME PLACES WHERE MOUNTAIN SICKNESS IS STUDIED

The study of mountain sickness owes much to the Italian physiologist Mosso. Mosso carried into this particular branch of physiology the tradition of the school to which he owed allegiance, that of Ludwig. To his enthusiasm and to his capacity to make that enthusiasm effective we owe the laboratory opened on the top of Monte Rosa[1] by Queen Margherita of Italy and called after her the Capanna Margherita.

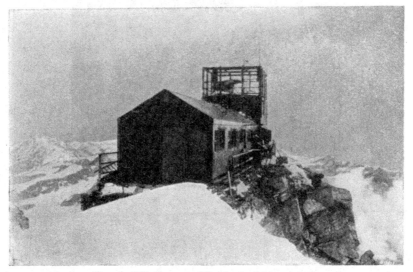

Fig. 4. The Capanna Margherita (Aggazzotti).

Let me leave the theoretical part of my discussion to say a few words about the Capanna Margherita and its surroundings. The altitude is about 5000 feet above the snow line. The summit is perched on a peak which is precipitous at one side, whilst on the other the

[1] Monte Rosa has several summits all of nearly the same height. The Punta Gnifetti on which the Margherita Hut is situated is not actually the highest, being within a few feet of 15,000. The highest peak is a much less accessible one, the Punta Dufour, 15,250 feet high.

ascent, though simple enough, consists for the last 1500 feet of a staircase of steps cut in the ice. Imagine a cone covered with ice. Imagine it to be bisected through the apex by a vertical cut, take away one half, that which remains is a tolerable representation of my recollection of the Punta Gnifetti. On the very top of this half cone and occupying the whole top is the Margherita Hut.

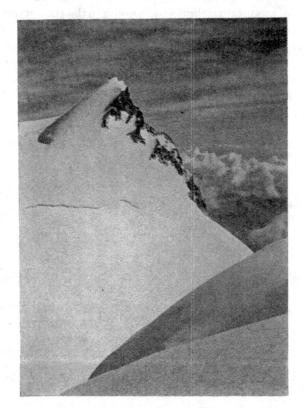

Fig. 5. The Punta Gnifetti on the summit of which is seen the Capanna Margherita (Durig).

The Hut consists of three compartments: the laboratory, with its small work rooms and sleeping room, secondly, the Alpine hut proper for the use of climbers, and thirdly, the portion which I believe belongs to the Italian army and is for the purpose of making meteorological observations.

Practical experience showed that the conditions at the Capanna Margherita are too rigorous. Although the hut itself is roomy and comfortable enough, the difficulty of transport greatly restricts the possibilities both of research and gastronomy. If you order a cup of hot coffee, for instance, the amount of spirit required to boil the water has to be considered. Spirit is the only fuel up there, much more of it is required to heat the water than at ordinary altitudes, and it all has to be carried up by porters. Note that I say "heat" not "boil," the water boils at about 180° F. Delicate or bulky apparatus is practically out of the question and even if it were not for these practical drawbacks, the low temperature and the confinement introduce factors which greatly complicate the effects of low atmospheric pressure.

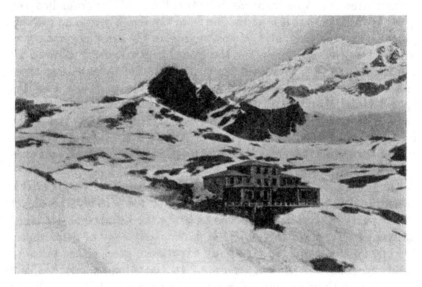

FIG. 6. The laboratory at Col d'Olen (Aggazzotti).

For these reasons the laboratory at Col d'Olen was founded. It is on the Italian face of Monte Rosa at an altitude of about 10,000 feet. In summer it is therefore just below the snow line and that is where a laboratory for the study of altitude should be, but the snow line is only high enough for about two months in the year to make much work there possible. I think the Col d'Olen laboratory is open only from about July 10 to Sept. 1. During that time it is well supplied with such of the comforts of life as can be brought thither on mules from Alagna or Gressoney and the amenities of the place are greatly enhanced by the skill and kindness of Professor Aggazzotti. There is water and there is gas, though at that altitude the gas flame is so attenuated as to give out a disappointingly small quantity of heat. But though, relatively to the snow line, Col d'Olen is properly situated in July and August, absolutely it is at too low an altitude. I do not think high altitude work is worth doing at a much lower altitude than 14,000 feet. Witness the controversy which used to exist as to whether the increase in red blood corpuscles wrought by altitude was a *bona fide* phenomenon. There could never have been any such controversy in the Andes or I suppose at Pike's Peak.

Such then are the advantages and the drawbacks of the best mountain station in the Alps. Let us pass to the Peak of Teneriffe.

To British or American workers the Peak of Teneriffe has the great advantage that it is accessible from the sea. There is no railway journey, no changing, and, if others receive the same hospitality as we did, no custom house, for the Spanish government allowed all our baggage to pass without being unpacked. For these reasons most of the apparatus arrived at the base intact. We made our base the Grand Hotel Humbert at Orotava. It was then in German hands, very comfortable, and we received every attention. How it may be now I do not know. The steamers of Troward Brothers go actually to Orotava from Liverpool; otherwise the traveller goes to Santa Cruz and drives to Orotava.

The island of Teneriffe has the advantage of a very equable climate. It is neither too hot, too cold nor too windy. The object of our party in working there was to study the human subject when at rest. In Teneriffe this object is particularly easy of attainment. No one on the island, so far as my experience goes, either takes or wants to take any violent exercise. In the Alps no one has any other object than exercise in some form or other, but to walk up the Peak of Teneriffe would be only less peculiar than to make the ascent to Col d'Olen on a mule.

Our sea-level station then was at Puerto Orotava. The "Humbert" was perhaps 300 feet above the sea-level; the climate when we were there, which was in March, was much like that of the English summer and was cool compared with that which we subsequently encountered at the sea-level station of our Italian expedition—Pisa.

The second station in Teneriffe was at Las Cañadas. From the point of view of the meteorologist this station is of especial interest. It is about 7000 feet above the sea-level and therefore not much higher than many centres of population—Johannesburg, for instance, is close upon 6000. Putting aside therefore such places as the mining towns in the Andes, the Cañadas is a fair example of the higher altitudes at which the working life of man is carried out on a normal scale. As a station for the study of climate the Cañadas can offer among other advantages, a relative immunity from wind. This, in view of the investigations published by Lyth (1), is a factor worthy of consideration.

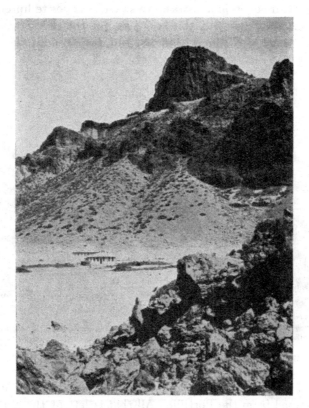

FIG. 7. The Cañadas showing the living house and the laboratory Espigone, one of the summits on the lip of the old crater in the background. View looking in the opposite direction from Fig. 1, which shows the "new crater."

The island of Teneriffe consists roughly of a huge crater about 8000–9000 feet in height. The diameter from lip to lip is eight miles. On the south side of the island the lip is incomplete. The inside of the lip is a steep, not quite precipitous, cliff, down which you must climb for a thousand or two feet, unless you enter the crater as we did by a gap in the cliffs called the Portillio. We were then inside the old crater; our back was to the cliff, which in places rises in named summits, Guajera and Espigone for instance. Our faces were towards a level plateau of sand.

From the description I have given so far it might be supposed that a sandy plain now stretched before our eyes, and that in the distance, six or seven miles away, we saw the opposite lip of the old crater in front of us. But this is not so, for the new crater, which had been thrust up from within the old, intervened; the majestic

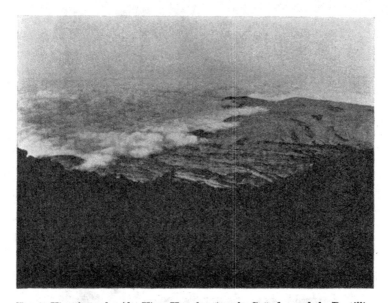

Fig. 8. View from the Alta Vista Hut showing the Cañadas and the Portillio.

Peak itself rising to an altitude of 12,000 feet burst suddenly upon us as we emerged from the Portillio. All that is left of the plateau is a ring of level sand in close proximity to the almost vertical lip of the old crater, on the outside of this ring rise the cliffs to about 1000 feet in height, on the inside the gradual ascent of the Peak. It was on this sand that our station was placed. No place at this altitude could have been more sheltered by natural barriers. It was quite unlike any place to be seen in Europe. Compared with much higher altitudes in the Alps, the comparison is a very remarkable one. The complete dryness of the atmosphere at the Cañadas accounts for the lack of the beautiful vegetation which makes the Alpine snow line so attractive. Go out of the laboratory at Col d'Olen; everything is moist underneath your feet, the cracks in the rock are filled with saxifrages and gentians. Not so at the Cañadas; the vegetation at low altitudes in Teneriffe is no less beautiful than in the Alps. To get to the Portillio one must ride through woods of giant heath which rise seven or eight feet into the air and burst into blossom above the head. But moisture condenses into clouds which hang over the island in a sheet at an altitude of 4000–5000 feet—through these clouds one penetrates. Once arrived within the old crater a new climate has been reached. Between one and the clouds there is an impassable rampart. No vestige of mist was seen either above us or around us during our sojourn in Las Cañadas, the occasional appearance of a cloud-top above the lip of the crater was the only reminder that such a thing as a cloud existed. Above the clouds all is barren.

The quarters at the Cañadas were quite comfortable; they consisted of two huts, made of some metallic composition, one of which was used as a living house and the other served as a laboratory. These huts, which were much larger and more substantial than the army hut with which we have since become so familiar, were reputed to be the property of the German Emperor. However this may be I do not know, at all events they were the domicile of a German meteorological organisation over which Herr Wenger presided. Our party, which styled itself the "International Commission for the study of high climate and solar radiation," had its origin in Berlin, it was stage-managed in the most efficient and at times sumptuous way by Prof. Pannwitz and was led by that physiologist of great insight Prof. Zuntz. It is probable that solar radiation and other climatic factors may be studied much more in the future than in the past. If so there may be a future for the Cañadas. It has a wonderful climate, though too low to be of much real service as a high altitude station, and close to the huts is one very important asset, namely, a spring of water. I hesitate to make any statement as to whether this is or is not the highest spring on the island. I saw none at any higher altitude.

Our high altitude station in Teneriffe was the Alta Vista Hut. It was situated at a level just short of 11,000 feet and just above the white patch which looks like snow on photographs of the Peak but is in reality pumice. At the time of year when I was there, April, there was no snow on the Peak and therefore, unlike the summit of Monte

Rosa, one could get about to any extent desired, but alternatively there is no accommodation for work. Apart from the shelves on which one may sleep, and a table and two chairs, all three decrepit, I remember but one piece of furniture. It was a stove which bore the label "Perfection"—I have lived to discover that the "Perfection" stove has great merits, but the particular article which confronted me at the Alta Vista fell further short of its name than almost anything I have ever seen. Let me remind you that not only had it to be used for cooking and for heating the hut, but for the very im-

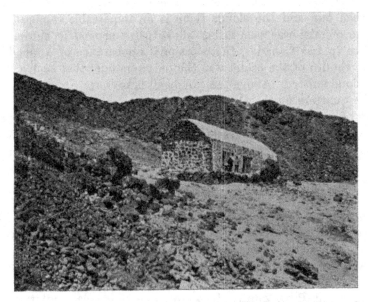

Fig. 9. The Alta Vista Hut, 11,000 feet. Standing near the door and dressed in black is the late Professor Zuntz.

portant function of melting ice. The sole supply of this precious material is a cave from the interior of which the ice may be hewn, situated about ten minutes' walk from the Alta Vista Hut.

Having now had to do with the planning of four mountaineering expeditions I have come to regard laboratory accommodation in a rather curious light. The places in which I have worked divide themselves into three categories. Firstly, those in which you can get both hot and cold water—such are hotel bathrooms. Secondly, those in which you can get cold water but not hot, such are the laboratories of Col d'Olen on Monte Rosa at about 11,000 feet and the Cañadas in Teneriffe at 7000 and, lastly, such places as the Alta Vista and the Margherita Hut at which if you require water you must make it by the laborious process of melting ice. In other words the classification of these places in my own mind tends to be less one of altitude than one of temperature.

I have dwelt for a moment on what may seem to be comparative trivialities for the purpose of impressing you with something which is by no means trivial, and which I shall proceed to put to you. It is the essence of well conceived scientific work that only one variable should be changed at a time. If that variable is to be altitude, then in all other respects the experiments at high and low altitudes should be under similar conditions. Supposing therefore I make comparative tests on the human frame say at Pisa and the Capanna Margherita or at Orotava and the Alta Vista Hut, how am I to know that what I observe on the height is in reality the effect of rare air and not the effect of cold? The ideal is to find two places with much the same temperature, one at say 15,000 or 16,000 feet altitude the other at the sea-level. Such of course cannot be found in close proximity but there are a few suitable places in the tropics which at this altitude have climates not unlike those of our homes in winter time. The two most obvious places of this character are the Himalayas in the Old World and the Andes in the New. Nor does this question of variables end with cold and altitude. It is impossible to lead any kind of normal life at the Capanna Margherita because of the difficulties of transport and the confined nature of the place. Most people who stay there for any length of time find that their digestions go very much astray. In fact they become quite poorly, sometimes it is diarrhœa, sometimes it is the reverse. But is it certain that the cause is altitude, or even cold? If you do not get any proper food what is likely to be the result? And if your digestion goes wrong how many of the other ills from which you suffer are merely secondary to the indigestion? It is therefore most desirable that work at high altitudes should be carried on at the sort of place where normal people lead a normal life; where the ordinary amenities of civilisation, such as properly cooked and served meals, proper sleeping accommodation and the proper amount of exercise may be obtained. Of such places two have been used for researches of importance, namely, Pike's Peak in Colorado and Cerro de Pasco in Peru.

Of Pike's Peak I would like to be able to speak at first hand but alas I cannot. Its height, 15,000 feet, is about the same as that of the Capanna Margherita, in summer it is near the snow line, it affords every necessary comfort as tourists make the ascent in large numbers during the milder parts of the year. Its accessibility to the ever increasing number of physiologists in the United States and Canada will always insure a large amount of work being carried out there. Moreover, there is a railway to the summit so that it fulfils the general conditions indicated in the preceding chapter as a

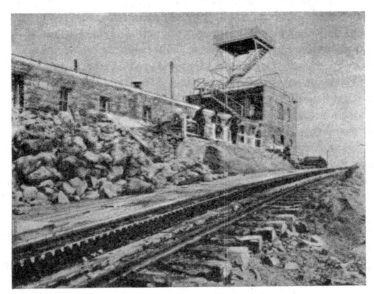

Fig. 10.   Pike's Peak observatory, Colorado, altitude 14,000 feet (Haldane, Douglas, Henderson and Schneider).

place in which to study oxygen deficiency, relatively uncomplicated by other factors.

If the reader should ever make use of these pages for the purpose of selecting a station at which himself to work he must recollect that in comparing Pike's Peak with the mining districts of the Peruvian Andes, I am comparing a place where I have not been to one with which I am acquainted, and probably more than a touch of prejudice enters the comparison.

Apart then from the expenditure of time and money necessary to reach Cerro de Pasco, it seems to me to have certain great advantages over Pike's Peak. Firstly, and least important, is the fact that one

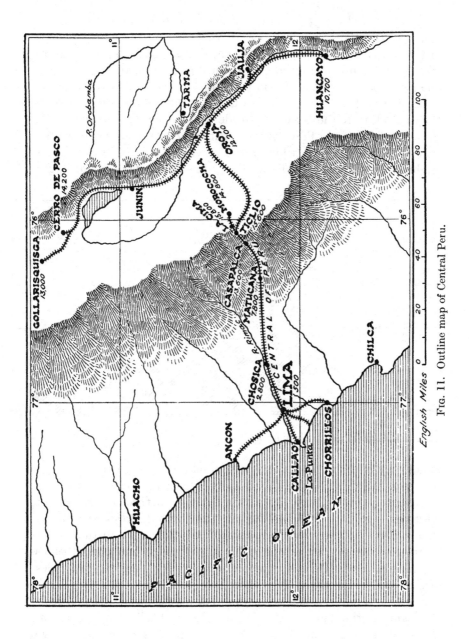

Fig. 11. Outline map of Central Peru.

can get to it from the sea-level within a day. Cerro itself is some 80 miles beyond Oroya and this takes about four hours in the train, which leaving Callao about 6–7 a.m. arrives at Cerro about 9 o'clock in the evening, but as has already been indicated, the train reaches the highest point on the line, at about 3 p.m. so that in nine hours one may ascend almost 16,000 feet by rail. Secondly, and directly connected with the first point, is the fact that whereas the hotel at Pike's Peak is at the highest altitude in the vicinity it is easy from the central railway of Peru to reach altitudes considerably higher than that of Cerro de Pasco, which in an extended series of experiments might serve as a sort of base. Cerro itself is a valley, one might

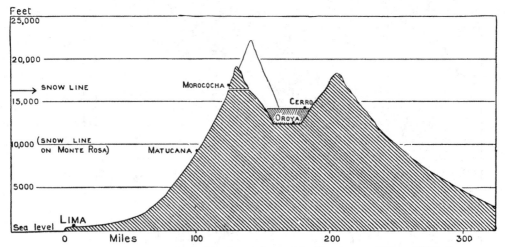

Fig. 12. Profile diagram to show altitudes of places visited by the expedition of 1921–2.

almost say in a cup, but it is a broken cup, for there is an outlet at one point through which the railway leaves for Oroya. The hills immediately round Cerro, i.e., within a couple or three miles, are not very high—perhaps 1500 feet higher than Cerro itself so that just in that vicinity I think there is no land of 16,000 feet in altitude. But there are other mining camps of less importance where the altitudes run higher. From Ticlio a branch line leaves for a camp a few miles distant called Morococha, here there is quite a considerable organisation and I think the houses in this district run up to 16,000 feet. The same is the case a little further down the line at Casapalca. The smelter itself is at a lower level, but there is a mine shaft above it which opens at about 16,000 feet altitude. In all this district, i.e.,

Ticlio, Morococha and Casapalca the summits of the mountains are very fine and are between 17,000 and 18,000 feet in altitude. The highest which our party attained was Mount Carlos Fernandez, the ascent of which we made from Casapalca, guided by our good friends and hosts, Mr Colley and Mr Campbell. Another place at which it might be possible to work would be "the Vanadium mine," which can be reached easily from Cerro de Pasco. This, I believe, is also about 16,000 feet altitude.

I must not proceed without some further mention of the kindness with which our party were met at every point in our visit to Peru; indeed to say that we owed such success as we achieved very largely to the kindness of those with whom we came in contact would be seriously to understate our indebtedness. I shall make no attempt here to catalogue our benefactors, the reader will learn something of what we owe them if he peruses the following pages.

I have enumerated various places within perhaps 150 miles of one another and more or less on the Central Railway of Peru as being suitable for high altitude research, and this fact alone brings me to the question of transport. Now one of the great advantages of the Andes was insured to us by the hospitality of the Central Railway, who gave us a full-sized luggage van, or, as it is called in America, a "baggage car," which we converted into a laboratory, and also a covered truck or "freight car" for our stores. The full meed of their generosity was apparent when we came to some of the steeper levels— gradients of 1 in 20—for there a freight car and a baggage car constituted a great proportion of a whole train. How sumptuous this laboratory as compared with the Alta Vista Hut—how convenient as compared with the Capanna Margherita! It could be taken to any place on the railway system and could therefore form a base for work at any altitude which that part of the Andes offers; at any station where there is a smelter electric current was available, and therefore we had the car heated by electricity, we had electric power, and we could run an X-ray apparatus. How different from the gas at Col d'Olen which went out at the critical moment, or the "Perfection" stoves in Teneriffe! A baggage car 45 feet in length forms a good and comfortable laboratory, and when in addition one can take it to any locality from the sea-level to 16,000 feet—well, what more can be desired? The car had, however, to be fitted up for its purpose. That was largely accomplished before my arrival in Peru. The American members of my party—Redfield, Bock, Binger, Forbes and Harrop arrived at Lima about three weeks before Meakins, Doggart and myself, the interval they spent in fitting up the laboratory. Benches were put all round, the space occupied by the great sliding doors on one side was filled in up to the level of the bench and a window placed above. Little had to be done in the way of fitting cupboards. There were shelves up in the roof which held innumerable smallish articles. This orgy of carpentry was carried out by carpenters kindly placed at our disposal by the Grace Line. Armed with a mobile laboratory which "would go anywhere or do anything"—on the railway—we set off "up the hill" on December 19, 1921.

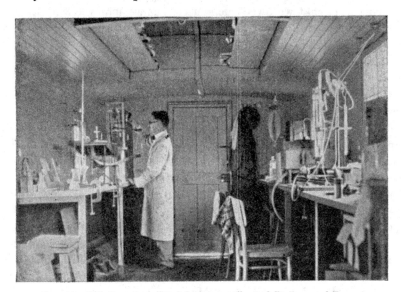

FIG. 13. Interior of mobile laboratory, Central Railway of Peru.

So far as "hotels" go, I think there are only two institutions which would suggest that word between Lima and Oroya. These are at Chosica and Matucana. The hotel at Chosica is quite good. Chosica itself is a resort with a "season," at an altitude of about 2000 feet, and is therefore at too low a level to be of use even for purposes of acclimatisation. Matucana possesses a good hotel, but "good" according to a different standard from that at Chosica. The Chosica hotel is good, among other reasons, because one may find no fleas in one's bed. The Matucana hotel is to be judged by the relative, but not invariable, absence of something else. But life in the Matucana hotel is quite pleasant if you are prepared to rough it a little. For my part I look back to the Railway hotel at Matucana with a feeling of warm affection, for within its precincts I had a night's sleep so profound and satisfying as to form a land-mark in my visit to South America. It was the night of our ascent of Carlos Fernandez—our last effort in high mountains. From about 17,500 feet in five hours I had descended to 7700. The descent of the first 1000 or 1500 feet made by the exhilarating process of sliding down on the snow, then 3000 feet on horseback, and for the remaining 6000 feet we reverted to gravity as a means of propulsion, but this time on a four-wheeled bogie in which we rattled down the railway. I do not know whether it was due to the return to a more normal oxygen pressure, or to the sudden lifting of the strain necessarily incident to the direction of the expedition, or to the reaction after three weeks of fretful sleep, or to all three reasons combined, but, be the cause what it may, I slept round the clock at Matucana and with sleep of such quality as to make the night one long to be remembered.

And now to return to our consideration of the merits of Peru, and especially its merits relative to Pike's Peak. I must say something about the amenities of life at Cerro de Pasco. The Peruvian Consul in London, Mr Victor Oscar Salamon, to whom I owe much, prepared me for Cerro by saying somewhat jocularly: "If the Cerro de Pasco Company make you their guests you will have a dinner as good as the Ritz every evening," and that was near enough to the truth to give the correct impression of what their kindness meant. Four of us were housed in a cottage, but it was a cottage which possessed a bath-room and any amount of hot water, two comfortable bed-rooms, a sitting-room with a fine fire-place and a kitchen in which we stored our baggage. The rest were housed in the Club, where we all had our meals.

The Club was a large one-story building disposed round a square; each pair of bed-rooms had a bath-room and lavatory attached; these constituted the quarters of the unmarried members of the Cerro de Pasco Corporation staff. The married ones lived in such little houses as the one I have just described.

Fancy the vision which must have arisen before the eyes of the staff at Cerro when they heard that eight men of science were coming amongst them to carry out researches. To the Cerronians the prospect must have been that of individuals who would present the greatest possible contrast to themselves. Now the Cerronians were men of great muscular strength and physical endurance, men who had roamed all over the American continent from Hudson's Bay to Patagonia, men who had been through every hardship and who lived chiefly for adventure, men wide in outlook and large in soul; if they imagined us as their antitheses then they must have looked for the advent of eight human beings, of the blue-spectacled and bearded variety, inferior in physique, inclined to grumble at discomfort and mentally enclosed in a groove of abstract scientific thought. Yet they welcomed us straight away, they were helpfulness itself from the start. Not only did they give us every facility for work, but socially they took us to their bosom, included us in their Christmas festivities which culminated on the last night of the old year, in a dance at "the Smelter" a few miles away. Here the whole community of the mining engineers of the Cerro de Pasco organisation was represented. Not merely the staff of the mines at Cerro itself, but officials, their wives and their people came from Oroya, from Morococha, from Casapalca, from Gollarisquisga and from other places which I only dimly remember, and at an altitude of about 13,000 feet we all danced in the new year, most of us in the literal sense. Four of our party, excepting a gap for supper, took the floor continuously from 9.30 p.m. till 2.30 a.m. at which time the proceedings terminated. About half-past three Meakins and I were making our way from the station at Cerro up to our cottage when he turned to me and said: "Many less remarkable physiological experiments have been performed than that."

Another great advantage which Cerro de Pasco possesses is the equability of its climate throughout the year. Col d'Olen is only open for about six weeks to two months. I do not know how it may be at Pike's Peak, but at Cerro the summer and winter temperatures do not differ greatly. We were there in the summer of the southern hemisphere. The climate then was like November in England. The Cerronian winter is, I believe, a little colder and a good deal brighter. In any case a research could be sustained at Cerro under not very unequal conditions of temperature the whole year round.

There remains to be discussed, Everest; which I take to be the extreme type of what it is—high, inaccessible, rigorous. It has but one advantage, namely, its height. Certain determinations can be made there which cannot be made elsewhere. Such must be of a primitive kind, and mostly without apparatus, but if you wish to get such information as may be had at the highest altitudes to which man can climb, there is but one place to go to, for he has achieved on Everest an altitude higher than that of any locality which exists outside Thibet.

BIBLIOGRAPHY

(1) LYTH.

CHAPTER III

THE DWELLERS AT HIGH ALTITUDES

In the preceding chapter I gave the more material reasons for the choice of Peru as the most suitable place for research on the physiological effects of high altitude. I said also that there was an additional reason for going there which transcended all the rest, namely, that living up in the Andean Pampa was an indigenous population, whose physiological processes afforded a field for study far superior to any which had hitherto been explored.

Let me turn to some description of these people and, without going into great detail, give some account of such peculiarities in their constitutions as may properly be attributed to the altitude at which they exist, or which may plausibly be discussed in that connection.

In describing the native of the mountains my first difficulty is to discover by what name he is to be designated. Almost any generic term which I might apply to him carries with it some assumption with regard to his ancestry and race which I should wish to avoid, and the validity of which I should like later to discuss. The term Peruvian, for instance, includes the descendants of the original Spanish settler, and indeed would by them be regarded as excluding the plebeian of Cerro de Pasco. The term Indian would probably be much more applicable, but not being an anthropologist I should hesitate to use it, and in any case it is clear that the rank and file of a population which has been in contact for centuries with races of European origin, as that of Cerro has done, cannot be regarded as pure-blooded. I shall therefore call the people by the vernacular word used to describe them up there in Peru, namely "Cholos." I do not know how far the term may be regarded as classical English, but I think it would be applied to any man who wears a poncho in any part of Peru. I use it merely to describe the man in the street of Cerro, excluding, on the one hand, his ruler of Spanish ancestry and, on the other, his employer of Anglo-Saxon parentage.

Our party made no further attempt to ascertain the nationality of Cholos on whom we worked than to find out their birth-place and to see that they were of the same general type as the rest of the indigenous population. Some future expedition will, I hope, so far improve upon our methods as to satisfy themselves of the pure-bloodedness of their victims—it might then be possible to draw some more satisfactory line between the effects of altitude on the race and its effects on the individual. All this, I think, could be done, but not in a short time, and of course would be eminently worth doing. To be reasonably sure that an individual was of the ancient stock it would be better to go outside Cerro de Pasco and seek material in the outlying villages. Not that any records are available to indicate the pedigrees of the inhabitants, but the customs of these villages remain so primitive as to suggest that the community in each has remained isolated from the influence of outside civilisation.

Not far from Gollarisquisga, the coal-mining centre of the Cerro Company, I was shown a number of such villages. In each of these the holding of property is communal. The farms radiate from the village in sectors of circles, and land in one or other of these sectors is assigned to the villagers to till. The produce is brought by each individual to the village for distribution. Money has no value to these people. Commodities are acquired by barter, not by the individual but by the community. If, for instance, coca is required and the village stock is exhausted, some one goes to a marketing centre such as Huancayo and acquires a new hoard for the village.

These customs, so far as I can make out—I speak, of course, entirely as a layman and can lay no claim to be an ethnologist—go back to days which precede not only the Spanish conquest of Peru by Pizarro but also the previous Inca civilisation.

Who the Incas were and whence they came I do not know, but, whoever they may have been, their arrival in Peru only antedated that of the Spaniards by about three centuries (1). They were numerous enough to impose their civilisation on considerable portions of Peru while their power lasted, but I think not numerous enough to produce any profound effect on the racial characteristics of the Cholo at a distance of four to five centuries. Their scheme however was not a purely communal one—under the Inca régime the produce of the country was divided into three portions, one-third only went to the community, of the remaining two-thirds, one went to the Church (not, of course, the Christian Church, for they were worshippers of the Sun) and the remaining third to the Inca or Chief.

If then the race has remained as true to type as to its customs, one may suppose that there will have been but little intermixture of blood in the village communities since pre-Incas days. To secure a syringe-full of such blood it would be necessary to win the confidence of a very shy population, which would however require time and patience, and I have little doubt from what I saw that it could be done, and one day I hope it will.

We however had to take the Cholo of Cerro as we found him, taking his word for it that he had been born and bred in the neighbourhood, and that being granted, we became more interested in his capabilities than in his pedigree.

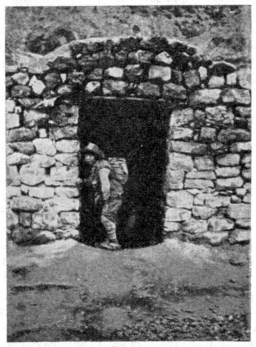

Fig. 14.

The Cholos are capable of performing feats of physical strength and endurance which are very surprising. A couple of examples may be given.

Cerro is a place of contrasts; close to some of the most perfectly operated mines that one can imagine there is an old mine operated by a Spaniard. In it the methods used have changed but little from those in vogue when Pizarro's immediate followers extracted silver from the neighbourhood of Cerro, though I believe not—as is sometimes stated—from the town itself. Fig. 14 shows the mouth of this mine. It looks like a small stone hut. Shortly after our arrival there a couple of little boys emerged, each with a load of ore on his back. One of the boys said he was but ten years of age. It is doubtful whether he knew to within three or four years what his age was, and we therefore place him at thirteen. The load of metal which he had carried from the bowels of the earth was about 40 lbs., the stone staircase up which he had carried it consisted rather of stumbling blocks than of stairs, its length was about 600 feet and its vertical height about 250 feet. Every few minutes like a bee out of some hive in cold weather, someone would appear from the mouth of the mine. He would be much out of breath, he would take frequent pauses on the way up, but the weight on his back would be a hundred pounds. Down he would put his weight, adding it to a pile composed of his previous loads for the day, down he would sit for a while to rest, and then down the mine again he would go to bring up another load. These porters, like a great part of the rest of the population, chew coca leaves, to this they attribute a part of their capacity for raising burdens. When the psychological moment for coca chewing arrives, nothing is allowed to interfere. The leaf of course contains cocaine. In contrast with such feats of endurance, and to bring out what they mean physiologically, let me put parallel to them our own experience. The incline from Cerro de Pasco railway station, where our laboratory was situated, to the Club was perhaps similar in gradient and length to that in London from the Houses of Parliament to the National Gallery or from the Rockefeller Institute in New York up Sixty-sixth Street. Before we left Cerro any of us could go up this with a fine swinging gait and with a semblance of respiratory comfort—so long as we were not burdened with an overcoat, but when the rain came on (as it did most afternoons at 3.30 unless a substitute appeared in the shape of snow) and we donned our trench coats, the progress was markedly slower and I will not say but that some of us stopped occasionally to take a long-drawn breath.

The second feat of physical endurance to which I would call attention is almost more remarkable. On one occasion, I think Christmas, it became necessary to erect a large cross some ten kilometres from the place at which it was made. The cross was of wood and I do not know what its weight may have been, but the photograph makes it quite clear that it must have been a burden which few ordinary persons would tackle even at the sea-level. Yet the Cholo carried this cross about seven miles over the country—and hilly country too—not walking, but at a jog-trot. The recent arrival can only sustain a walking pace, even if he has no burdens.

A very pleasant function was the dance to which the reader will find an allusion on page 36. I need only add here that the ladies with but few exceptions danced—apart from supper—the whole time during which the proceedings lasted. So you can dance in a partial vacuum (bar. 458) for about five hours and enjoy it thoroughly. But remember that it is all on the level. The ascent of Carlos Fernandez was a very different story. It was about 3000 feet higher up, but on the other hand we were much longer acclimatised. Those two facts may be held to cancel one another out. The ascent was for most of us a few steps and a pause, then another few steps, another pause and so on.

From Dr Kellas's manuscript I learn that the opinion which we had formed of the powers of endurance of natives when in high altitudes is not shared by many of those who have employed them. Humboldt seems first to have stated that they were less resistant than white men. In connection with his attempt on Chimborazo, he states that the Indians with one exception abandoned them at 15,600 feet, an altitude not much higher than Cerro. "Prayers and threats," says Humboldt, "were alike vain, they declared that they were suffering more than we." This view is corroborated by other Andean travellers such as Bouguer, whilst "Dr and Mrs Bullock Workman, Dr Longstaff and Sven Hedin have made similar statements regarding natives indigenous to from 8000 to 14,000 feet, but Dr Longstaff has also given the reason for this peculiar anomaly. He points out that the natives are as a rule carrying loads, which makes a great difference. Longstaff's observations agree with those of the author" (Kellas) "who has never observed a single case of mountain sickness in the case of picked trained natives climbing with him without loads in several expeditions to over 23,000 feet where clothing and food were carefully supervised."

Let us pass from the Cholo's capacity for sustained efforts to his physical characters. The Cholos are "a little people," little, that is to say, as far as height is concerned. Their faces are of a type which suggests Indian descent and their clothes the same. The hair is black and straight, the cheek bones are rather high, the nose is aquiline and the skin yellow. The hat is broad-brimmed, the body covered with a poncho; it is said that neither men nor women ever undress or wash. The last two statements I have not verified!

Two characteristics however he has which have a special interest for us as being possibly not racial but the direct result of the altitude at which he lives: one is the shape of his hands and the second that of his chest.

Fig. 15 represents a pair of hands which are quite typical examples of the extent to which the fingers are clubbed. Often the clubbing is much greater. The physician associated clubbing of the fingers with disorders of the circulatory and pulmonary system, which frequently are associated with oxygen want.

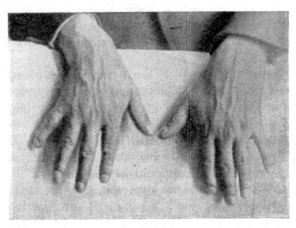

FIG. 15.

The feature about the Cholo however which I want most particularly to emphasise is the size and shape of his chest, which is large and especially deep, out of proportion to his stature.

The two differences between the Cholo and the European, which strike one most, are the colour of his face and the shape of his chest. The former we will treat with in another chapter, the latter demands consideration here for it is part of his physical development.

It is notorious amongst all visitors to the high Andes that many of the natives have large barrel-shaped chests which appear to be of great depth and give them somewhat the aspect of pouter pigeons. The question was treated statistically by Mr David Forbes (2) in 1870 in a paper published in the *Journal of the Ethnological Society* concerning which Sir Arthur Keith (3) comments that it "has provided the basis of all statements made regarding the great chest development of the Peruvians living on the high plateau. Many of Forbes' measurements were made by inexact methods and in several cases are manifestly erroneous." It was largely due to the stimulus of Sir Arthur Keith's interest in the matter that we made a considerable number of chest measurements of various sorts with which we shall now deal.

Our data are susceptible of certain generalisations which are of a quite superficial character: subsequent and independent analysis of them by Sir Arthur Keith and Dr Redfield brought out further facts, the consideration of which I shall defer till the end of the chapter. Let me deal now with the more obvious points of difference between the chest of the "Cholo" and that of the European or "Gringo."

We studied the chest in a number of ways, two of which I will discuss. They were by X-ray photography and by direct superficial measurement respectively. Firstly, then concerning the X-ray photographs. In Fig. 16 is shown the right halves of two photos, extending from the middle line outwards; that on the left-hand side is of a native and that on the right of one of our party. Here I should like to thank the General Electric Company and the Leeds and Northrup Company of Philadelphia for lending the field X-ray plant which it was our good fortune to have, and to Prof. Cannon who placed much of the accessory plant at our disposal. The contingencies of the war of course led to a wonderful advance in the possibilities of conducting X-ray research in relatively inaccessible places, and to this may be attributed the present introduction of the radiogram into anthropometric work. There is, of course, no inherent reason why the dimensions of people's insides should be less important than those of their outsides—simply they have not been measured for want of a proper method of measuring them. There was to me a very pleasing appropriateness about the fact that this innovation should have been made by Dr Redfield, at that time assistant to Prof. Cannon, just as twenty years ago Prof. Cannon himself was the pioneer in giving the X-rays an honourable place among the methods of physiological experiment. The first set of data which the X-ray films provided were those of the height and breadth of the chest respectively.

The height of the chest was taken to be the distance between the lowest point of the clavicle at its articulation with the sternum to the highest visible point on the diaphragm.

The breadth is that from the extreme point of the seventh rib on one side to that on the other.

The following table summarises these measurements and shows them in comparison with similar measurements obtained from the resident mining engineers and from ourselves. In the former case there were not enough data sufficient to average. The figures show that the height of the chest was markedly lower in the Cholos than in the white men but that the breadth in both cases was about the same.

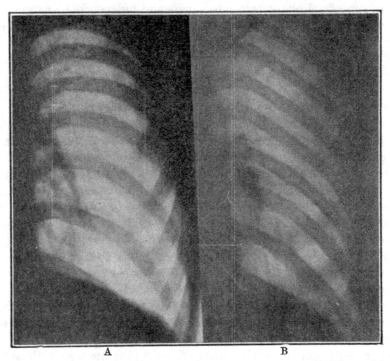

FIG. 16. Photos taken from behind. A, chest of native. B, chest of Barcroft.

Chest Measurements from X-ray Films

	Members of Expedition	Anglo-Saxon Residents	Indigenous Population
Height of chest	20–17·5 cm. Mean 18·5	20–18 cm. —	19·5–13 cm. Mean 15·7
Width of chest	28–26 cm. Mean 26·7	29–25·5 cm. —	28·5–23 cm. Mean 25·9

Such figures are however misleading for, as I said, the Cholos are a little people, while the engineers were persons of abnormally large physical development even for the white man, as also were our party, the average height of the engineers being five feet nine inches and that of our party five feet ten inches.

A truer comparison is to be obtained by dividing the chest measurement given above by the height of the body and multiplying the result by one hundred. The next table therefore gives the chest measurements as a percentage of the height of the body.

Mean Chest Measurements from X-ray Films
per 100 cm. of Height

	Members of Expedition	Indigenous Population
Height ...	10·4 cm.	10·2 cm.
Breadth ...	15 cm.	16·7 cm.

From the table it appears that relatively the height of the chest is the same in the Cholos and in ourselves, whilst the breadth of the chest was about 10 per cent. greater in theirs than in ours.

Somewhat the same story is told by the external measurements. In considering them we have the advantage of being able to compare the data obtained from the Cholos with the average of a vast number of measurements on Europeans and Americans accumulated by Prof. Dreyer, and in our work we have followed his system, i.e., we have taken the trunk measurement as the standard and compared the circumference of the chest with it.

Name	Occupation	Chest circumference calculated from trunk length	Chest circumference observed
B. C.	Carpenter	83·8 cm.	90·5 cm.
V.	Painter	74·1	82·5
A. O.	Lawyer	74·1	83·0
E. M.	Clerk	77·3	85·0
D. P.	Physician	83·2	81·0
G. R. A.	Merchant	83·8	92·0
F. V.	Blacksmith	84·9	95·0
F. M.	Book-keeper	77·9	87·5
P. J.	Waiter	82·2	82·2
Z.	Clerk	73·0	87·0
B.	Clerk	79·8	95·0
	Mean	79·8	87·3
Mean of 10 men at Morococha	Machinists or miners	79·2	92·3

The first column of figures shows what the chest measurement of an average Anglo-Saxon would be were his trunk length that of the Cholo in question. The second column shows what it actually was. The average calculated chest circumference for the first group of Cholos whom we measured was just under 80 cm., the average observed length was over 87 cm. These men were mostly persons of sedentary occupations, while the second group were manual workers, mostly machinists, and the disparity in their cases was even greater, the calculated chest circumference being 79·2 cm. and the observed being 92·3 cm.

Perhaps the most novel feature which a superficial examination

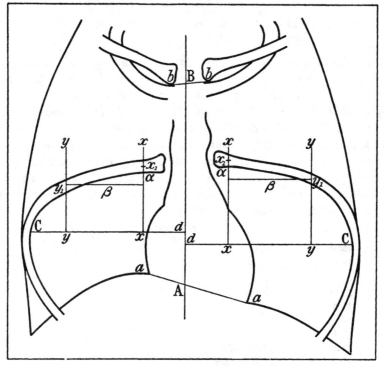

Fig. 17. (Redfield.)

of the X-ray photographs revealed, had reference to the position taken up by the ribs. In the Cholos the dorsal portions of the ribs are much more horizontally placed than in ourselves, as the mere inspection of the films shows. To give a numerical expression to the slope of the rib the following method was suggested to Dr Redfield. Let AB in Fig. 17 represent the mid-vertebral line. Cd is drawn from C perpendicular to the mid-line, the outermost point in the inner margin of the 8th rib. A similar line is drawn on the other side. Lines xx and yy are drawn parallel to the mid-line at distances

from it respectively of one-quarter and three-quarters the length
of Cd. The points x_1 and y_1 are located in xx and yy where these lines
cut the mid-line of the 8th rib. The slope of the rib may conveniently
be taken as the angle which a line joining x' and y' would make
with the horizontal. In the following data the slope given for the
individual is the average of that for his lower ribs.

In the case of our party the slope of the rib varied between 14·5
and 28 degrees to the horizontal, whilst the slope of the Cholo's ribs
varied between 6·5 and 22 degrees. The average values for the
Cholos was 13 degrees to the horizontal and for ourselves 21 degrees.

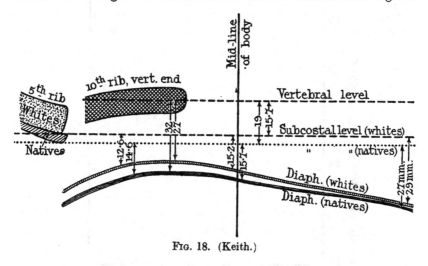

FIG. 18. (Keith.)

Let us turn to the more searching analyses of the films, taking
first that of Sir Arthur Keith [3] who very kindly went over all our
photographs on our return and added two main points with regard to
the natives. The first is that their diaphragms are less arched than
those of the Europeans, the second is that although the back of the
rib is more horizontal in the native than in the European, the front,
or sternal articulation which Prof. Keith was able to make out is
not higher. These points are shown in Fig. 18 in which the middle
of the vertebral end of the 10th rib is taken as a fixed point from
which measurements may be made, the highest point of the diaphragm
in the "whites" is 27 mm. below this line, that in the natives 32 mm.
below it. Just about the level of the vertebral articulation of the
10th rib may be seen faintly in the films the sternal articulation of
the 5th rib. This also Prof. Keith has transcribed on to the figure

showing that in the natives it ends almost in the same place—just a trifle lower than in the Europeans. Thus the rib of the native commencing and ending at approximately the same level as that of the European, but being much more horizontally disposed, really resembles more nearly the hoop of a barrel and gives a certain literal veracity to the "barrel-shaped" as applied to the chest of the Cholo.

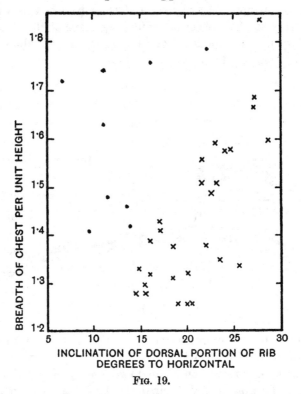

Fig. 19.

Dr Redfield's analysis is somewhat more complicated but it may be followed from Fig. 19.

In the preliminary analysis two points were mentioned: (1) the natives on the average had less sloping ribs at the back, (2) while the height of their chest was proportionately the same as that of the Anglo-Saxon's the breadth of the chest was proportionately greater. From which it follows that the breadth of the chest is greater relatively to the height of the chest in the natives than in the Anglo-Saxons.

In Fig. 19 the slope of the rib is placed horizontally. The crosses represent the ribs of our party and the dots represent the ribs of the natives. The slope which the selected portion of the rib makes with the horizontal plane is represented in degrees along the abscissa. Now it is clear that whilst on the average our ribs were more sloping than those of the natives, there were individual natives whose ribs sloped more than those of some of us, and therefore one could not be quite positive to which category a rib with a slope of 17 degrees belonged.

Similarly with the breadths of the chests that are plotted vertically. A chest which was precisely half as broad again, as it was high, and which therefore had a ratio of 1·5 on the ordinate might be an unusually narrow one for a native or an unusually broad one for a European.

The point which emerged from Dr Redfield's diagram, and it is in all essentials the same as Fig. 19, was that all the points contributed by the natives fall in an area that does not overlap, the area in which our points fall. One can therefore distinguish the chest of a native resident at Cerro from that of a European who has not been at so great an altitude for more than a few weeks by the comparison of an X-ray photograph of each. For some future worker there remains the problem of whether the difference is one which may be acquired by children whose bones are not set or even by adults, or whether on the other hand is it congenital? It is of interest in this connection to record that the natives dwelling at 14,000 feet in Thibet do not present the appearance of having unusually large chests, so Dr A. F. R. Wollaston tells me.

BIBLIOGRAPHY

(1) *Encyclopædia Britannica*, article "Peru."
(2) FORBES, D. *Journ. of Ethnological Soc.* New Series, 1870, vol. II. 193.
(3) KEITH, A. *Phil. Trans.* B. CCXI. 472. 1922.

CHAPTER IV

THE COLOUR OF THE FACE AND ITS SIGNIFICANCE

In the previous chapter, when speaking about the physical characteristics of the mountain dwellers, I made a passing reference to the
colour of their faces and said that I would reserve the matter for
future discussion. I do not mean, in using the phrase "the colour
of the natives" any allusion to whether they are a black, a white or
a yellow race, but my only concern is whether they are pale or
flushed, whether as the phrase runs "they have any colour in their
cheeks," and if so whether it is the fresh colour of a healthy person
or whether their cheeks are of a blue tinge such as is seen in middle-
aged or elderly persons suggesting heart pathology. Keen as was
our interest in the colour of the natives, we were at first almost
more concerned about our own. All the way up in the railway one
might have seen us examining the tint of the flesh beneath our finger-
nails. In this matter we were somewhat fortunate for accompanying
us was Dr Crane the Chief Medical Officer of the Cerro de Pasco
Company. He had come down from Oroya only two days before
and was on his way back. He therefore was a person thoroughly
acclimatised to life "on the Hill," and he formed an excellent
standard for comparison. It was evident that at any altitude from
8000 to 16,000 feet our finger-nails were bluer than his. This phenomenon has been noticed by many observers. The difficulty in its
interpretation heretofore has been that most of the previous ascents
have involved the transition from a warm to a cold climate, and that
therefore it has been difficult to know how much of the blueness of
the skin and nails has been due to cold and how much to deficiency
of oxygen in the blood. I remember on arrival at Col d'Olen calling
attention to the colour of my finger nails, only to be told that the
bluish tint was not the effect of altitude but of frost.

In Peru, however, there could be no question of that kind as we
went up to 15,800 feet in a heated car. Even so two facts were
apparent: firstly that all our nails and cheeks were bluer than at
sea-level and secondly that those of the party were bluer than those
of Dr Crane.

After two days' stay at Oroya the difference disappeared and our
nails were much like those of the doctor's, but in each case the
colour was not the same as at sea-level.

At Cerro de Pasco (14,000 feet) the abnormality of colour was more striking than at Oroya and was general, being obvious both amongst the residents of Anglo-Saxon extraction and the Cholos. Many of the latter were of a very ruddy appearance, but their cheeks were more a plum colour than a red. This is true even of the children.

In any interpretation of this phenomenon it must be borne in mind that these people have many more corpuscles in their blood than have normal people. Even down here such a person—a polycythæmic as he is called—has a typically bluish appearance, but there was abundant evidence that the colour was not due to the stagnant circulation of the polycythæmic but to a deficiency of oxygen in the blood. In the first place, if oxygen was given to such a person to breathe his face changed in colour in a matter of a few seconds, and in the second place, we had the opportunity of seeing the phenomenon disappear on descent from the "Hill" in a time so short that the number of corpuscles could not have been greatly changed. There was at Cerro an engineer whose cheeks were of a very high colour; on the mountains he had a purple, almost apoplectic appearance. Such a general appearance has been known to result from alcoholic excesses. He came down to Lima in the train with us, and when we saw him about half-way down quite a new vision burst on our eyes. Here was a man with the fresh, rosy complexion of a child, a man whose skin was so delicate that the colour conferred upon it by the blood in its capillaries was shown up to perfection. To say that he was a "cross between a chameleon and a barometer" would be undignified, so I shall avoid the phrase and adopt some more lengthy way of expressing my meaning which is that just as the chameleon passes through all the shades of one particular colour, say from light yellow to dark brown, or from light green through dark green to something nearly approaching black, so this man passed from a purple to a bright pink, the blue tinge which he had at Cerro becoming less and less accentuated with each thousand feet which he descended.

The plum colour which so readily came and went in the subject of whom I have spoken was a frequent feature in the aspect of the Cholos. Many of them were very sallow and ill-looking, having rather yellow skins unrelieved by any colour conferred by the blood, but where there was a flush it was of a plum colour which, combined with the pigment proper to the skin, gave them a rather browner appearance than that of our friend. The blue element in the colour of the capillary blood was best seen in the Cholo children. They had much more colour in their faces· than had their parents, and while it was always of a purplish tinge, one observed that the colour heightened and became more blue on physical exertion.

The reader may ask legitimately: "Why this concern about the colour of the Cholo?" Behind that there is a long story, which perhaps I had better tell from its commencement.

In the early nineties of last century work in industrial physiology was only at its commencement in England and indeed elsewhere. The pioneer in that line, and I imagine still the first authority on the subject, was Dr J. S. Haldane (1) of Oxford. He was then studying the effects of carbon monoxide in mine air and had been, not very long previously, a worker in the Physiological Laboratory at Copen-hagen then presided over by Professor Bohr. The fact about carbon monoxide which impressed Haldane was that in practice it was less fatal than was indicated by theoretical considerations.

Let me put the matter in this way. The hæmoglobin in a man's body is capable of combining with about a litre of carbon monoxide. The precise quantity necessary to kill him has, as far as I know, not been determined—let us say it is 700 c.c. Now suppose that a man enters a mine the· air of which contains a certain quantity of CO and exposes himself to it until his blood comes into equilibrium with it, each ounce of his blood will take up a certain amount; but if one draws an ounce of his blood and shakes it up with air corresponding to the man's alveolar air when in the mine, it will take up more CO than it actually does in the body. That at least was Dr Haldane's contention.

The question which Haldane put to himself was, if the CO does not get into the blood in the man's body in the calculated quantities, what keeps it out? He assumed that the properties of the blood itself are the same whether it be within or without the body. This assumption precluded any explanation along the lines of the blood having a greater affinity for carbon monoxide in the one case than in the other. If then less than the calculated quantity of CO was found in the blood, what kept the remainder out of it? The answer which Dr Haldane gave was that oxygen kept it out, and I must now try to explain how oxygen could accomplish this feat.

Of course both oxygen and carbon monoxide can combine with the hæmoglobin of the blood, but the affinity of the hæmoglobin for CO is 246 times that for oxygen, so that if you expose blood to an atmosphere which contains one million molecules of CO and 246 million molecules of oxygen, one half of the hæmoglobin will unite with the oxygen and the other half with the carbon monoxide (the same molecule of hæmoglobin cannot unite with both at the same time).

Suppose then that in the air of the lungs there are 240 molecules of oxygen for each molecule of carbon monoxide one might then expect that in the arterial blood half the hæmoglobin would be united with oxygen and half with carbon monoxide. If this is not the case, if less than half of the hæmoglobin is united with CO and more than half with oxygen it is clear that the oxygen must have some sort of "pull" over the CO. This "pull" according to Haldane was supplied by the epithelium of the lung which actively seized the oxygen in the air of the alveoli and actually thrust it through the body of the cell itself and into the blood, so that a more rapid stream of oxygen penetrated the lung-wall than would have been the case had the gas simply gone through the wall by a process of diffusion. In this way the pressure of oxygen inside the lung wall was increased to more than 246 times that of the carbon monoxide, the person therefore would have correspondingly less of his hæmoglobin associated with CO and correspondingly more with oxygen.

This alleged power of the epithelium of the lung cell to "pull" or "push" or "suck" or "thrust" or "secrete" oxygen through its substance into the blood has been a subject of continual speculation by physiologists, ever since the experiments of Haldane were published. The theory itself was first put forward by Professor Bohr (2) but on quite insufficient evidence, and Haldane's observation gave it its first substantial support. The importance of the theory lies in the fact that such a faculty, were it possessed by the lung, would be the cardinal phenomenon exhibited by that organ.

The efficiency of the lung would depend upon whether this secretory power were at its best or were impaired, just as the efficiency of the stomach depends upon whether the secreting cells are producing gastric juice in adequate quantities and of a proper degree of peptic activity. In all diseases of the lung the first question which would arise would be, are the cells secreting properly and if not how can they be stimulated to do so? For my own part I only took rather an academic interest in the matter until I was brought face to face with it during the war, in connection with the subject of gas poisoning. It did not matter from what angle of gas warfare the question was approached, no clear conception could be formulated until the question of whether the lung did or did not secrete oxygen was settled.

I will now approach the problem from the angle at which I first came in contact with it. During the days immediately after the first German gas attack several scientific men were summoned to France from England, myself among the number. The particular question which was put to me by Sir John Bradford was as to how the gas had affected its victim and amongst the first patients whom I saw, at the Base was one man whom I have never forgotten. His face, as he sat propped up in bed, was not in any way remarkable in colour, but on making the very slightest effort his colour changed. A purplish tinge appeared, which commencing at his ears gradually spread over his whole face, until he was what doctors would call markedly cyanosed.

Were Dr Haldane's hypothesis correct the probable explanation of this man's condition would have been that the gas had affected the power of his lungs to secrete the oxygen through the epithelium and hence that a forced pressure of oxygen which should have been established in the blood was not established. That the man was suffering from a sort of pulmonary dyspepsia. And so with regard to many other pulmonary complaints. If the physical factors involved are to be discussed in any quantitative way one must be clear that they are not all being masked by another factor, namely, that of oxygen secretion.

The study of gas poisoning, and a number of other conditions during the war, brought the question of the quantity of oxygen in the arterial blood into great prominence. In the early days of the war it was only possible to guess the extent to which the arterial blood was saturated with oxygen, towards the end of the war a technique was developed for its measurement.

The difficulty which had existed was that of obtaining the blood from an artery. This difficulty was solved by Dr Stadie(3), from the Rockefeller Institute in New York, who devised the method known as that of arterial puncture. The point of a hypodermic needle is thrust through the skin right into the radial artery and the blood is withdrawn into a syringe attached to the needle.

In this way it became possible to make numerous analyses of the arterial blood of men. The results which were very constant in normal persons showed that the blood was always of a bright red colour and contained 95–96 per cent. of the maximal quantity of oxygen which it could theoretically carry.

An important school of thought then arose which held that something must be seriously amiss with a subject if the oxygen in his blood deviated by more than one per cent. or so from the 95–96 per cent. standard. One heard of anoxæmia—or insufficient oxygen in the blood—on all sides. It was found also that in many conditions such as that of pneumonia there was a very marked anoxæmia, instead of the blood being 95–96 per cent. saturated it was perhaps only 80 per cent. (4) saturated and the question naturally arose to what extent the patient was being poisoned by the toxic products of the pneumococcus bacillus and to what extent he was only being asphyxiated by the want of oxygen in the blood. I say "only" because the latter condition can be met largely by the administration of oxygen to the patient. It became a very important medical question. The piece of information necessary to its solution was whether a similar degree of anoxæmia could be induced in a normal person, and if so, whether the person would remain normal or would be in a condition of semi-asphyxiation.

The information might appear at first sight easy to obtain. It might seem that the pressure of oxygen need only be reduced in the lungs to the point at which the blood would cease to be 95–96 per cent. saturated with the gas and the saturation of the blood would commence to fall. But just at this point Dr Haldane's theory baffled argument. Haldane's (4) position when he published *Organism and Environment* was expressed in the following words: "The mean result was that on Pike's Peak after acclimatisation, the arterial oxygen pressure was during rest about 13 mm. lower than at sea level, but was 35 mm. higher than the alveolar oxygen pressure. The complete absence of any blueness after acclimatisation was early intelligible. The lungs were actively secreting oxygen into the blood, even during rest. Nevertheless the blueness reappeared temporarily during prolonged muscular exertion as in a long climb. The lung epithelium could thus apparently be fatigued by the extra work thrown upon it."

He said in effect, only temporarily can you produce more than a trivial change in the pressure of oxygen in the blood. The argument was that deduced from his experiments on carbon monoxide poisoning. He held that if you try to reduce the percentage of oxygen in the blood in that way you will discover that the epithelial cells of the lung tissue will defeat you. They will take what oxygen there is, and they will secrete it by main force through the epithelial wall, causing it to arrive in the blood at the normal pressure, and saturate it up to the normal saturation. He laid down the principle in fact, that the essential property of the lung cell was just that. It delivered oxygen at a definite pressure of approximately 100 mm. of mercury into the blood, and saturated up to 95 per cent. whatever the oxygen in its environment might be. Nor was this mere speculation. On Pike's Peak (5) a party of scientists, of whom Dr Haldane was the chief, carried out a number of experiments by extremely complicated methods, in which their published figures were entirely in agreement with the line of thought indicated above. For after a short residence there, the pressure of oxygen in the blood appeared to be about 90–110 mm. in spite of the fact that the pressure of oxygen in the air of the lungs was but 50 mm., or thereabouts.

It is seen therefore that there are two main points at stake: (1) The philosophical point—namely, whether the living cell does exercise this control.

We will now discuss Dr Haldane's philosophic position. He further took up the attitude that this property was the essential manifestation of the life of the cell, that it was its identity, that its individuality consisted in controlling its environment in just this way. That if one said "you" to the lung cell, one was addressing an identity which found its power of self-expression in turning a continually varying oxygen pressure which it found on its alveolar side into a constant oxygen pressure of 100 mm. which it discharged on its capillary side. If one asked what controlled the cell in this matter there was no answer. Its existence consisted not in being controlled but in controlling—that was its "ego." (6) And this principle was extended to other cells in the body. The "ego" of the kidney cell was to control the amount of water in the blood and so forth.

(2) The medical point, namely, whether in the event of the cell in the pulmonary epithelium being unable to control the pressure of oxygen in the blood, or in the event of its losing such control, would the patient suffer, and if so, how much?

At times I have heard persons speak as though there was some inherent absurdity in Haldane's theory and as though it were intellectually unworthy of the great man who pinned his confidence to it. Up to the point to which I have brought the reader let me convince him that I am quite out of sympathy with such statements. It seems to me to be a very good theory. The demand which it makes on the cells of the pulmonary epithelium is one with which we are familiar in other cells of the body, namely, that they achieve something at the expense of a transformation of energy within their own substance. The necessary expenditure is quite trifling, as has been calculated by A. V. Hill(7), and the end is eminently worth while. Moreover, there occur cases in the animal kingdom in which certain cells in the lung can do something rather analogous—they can take oxygen from the blood and excrete it into the lung, this takes place in the swim bladder of fishes. Of course that is no real argument for or against the secretion of oxygen from the human lung, but it is evidence that the conception is not absurd. The question in my mind when Haldane's theory took the form, which I have described, was not whether the theory was a good one, but whether it was really supported by the facts. I determined that when the war was over I would put the matter to a direct test and avoiding all round about methods, secure blood directly from an artery after a residence of a considerable length of time, say a week, in an atmosphere poor enough in oxygen materially to reduce the percentage saturation of that gas in arterial blood should no secretion take place. That experiment needs but brief comment; it was carried out, over six days the pressure of oxygen in my respiration chamber was reduced to one which corresponded to about 18,000 feet at its lowest and which stood at about 15,000 feet when the crucial test was made. Arterial blood was withdrawn from a cannula in the radial artery and the saturation tested. Into the precise figures I need not go, the colour of the blood was enough. Never I suppose will curiosity rise in me to a higher pitch than it did at the moment before the clip on my artery was liberated and the blood allowed to flow. Was it to be the colour of ordinary arterial blood or was it to be perceptibly venous in appearance? The event left no doubt, it was dark; and more than this, when the necessary samples had been taken and I commenced to breathe an atmosphere rich in oxygen, the blood immediately flashed out red and a last sample taken after but twenty seconds of oxygen respiration was fully saturated.

A week's acclimatisation, or at all events a week's exposure to low oxygen pressure had apparently done nothing to make my lung secrete. I gather that Haldane himself carried out a similar experiment subsequently; I know but few details of it other than are disclosed in the meagre account in his book (8). It would seem that the result was much the same as that of my own experiment; and in both cases I am sure the colour of our faces and especially of our lips told the same tale as that of our arterial blood.

If the lung could not be tempted to secrete by about a week's residence in an oxygen pressure, which at the end was lower than that of the highest Alpine summit, there remained the possible criticisms: (1) that I was not as other men and that my lung was too poor a representative of its class to react to the stimulus of anoxæmia; (2) that life was too restricted and unnatural in a respiration chamber to enable the organism to react as it would, and as Haldane alleged that it did, on Pike's Peak.

The answer to both these criticisms was to be found in the Andes. The younger and more athletic members of our own party might be expected to accommodate as easily as the average of mankind. The lungs of the mining engineers would surely secrete if those of any white man could and emphatically in so far as acclimatisation to high altitudes is possible, one might expect to find it in the natives of the plateau, whose ancestors have, as would appear from their customs, been there for over 800 years.

The above summary, necessarily brief[1], will enlighten the reader as to our anxiety to note every passing change of colour in ourselves and in one another as we ascended the Central Railway of Peru, to compare our own cyanosis with that of Dr Crane who was thoroughly acclimatised, and finally to observe the colour in the cheeks of the Cholos.

The cyanosed appearance of the more delicate surface of the body is but a reflection of the condition of the blood. By using the technique devised by Dr Stadie of the Rockefeller Institute in New York, we were able to get samples of our own arterial blood for analysis. Not only so, but the mining engineers at Cerro entered into our doings with wonderful goodwill and offered themselves to us as victims, the native Cholo population with a little inducement followed their example. We therefore had the opportunity of testing the condition of the arterial blood in three classes of persons who were acclimatised in varying degrees, the Cholos whose ancestors had probably been in the hills for generations, the engineers who had

[1] A more complete account of the history of thought on this subject, up to 1914, will be found in *The Respiratory Function of the Blood*, Cambridge, 1914. Chapters XII and XIII.

been there for months or years, and ourselves whose period of acclimatisation could only be counted in days, or at most weeks.

Yet in each category the same striking condition of the arterial blood was evident, as soon as the needle of the hypodermic syringe was thrust into the radial artery and the blood commenced to force its way into the barrel it was evidently different in colour from ordinary arterial blood, instead of being bright red it was dark in appearance, more or less simulating the colour of venous blood.

The interpretation of the change in colour was, of course, not far to seek. The hæmoglobin of the blood did not contain its full load of oxygen. If normal blood be shaken up with oxygen the hæmoglobin present will unite with 1·34 c.c. of oxygen for each gram of the pigment which is present. Normal arterial blood, i.e. blood exposed not to air but to the poorer oxygen mixture which exists in the lung, contains 96 per cent. of this amount and we call it 96 per cent. saturated (or sometimes 4 per cent. unsaturated). The blood at Cerro de Pasco fell far short of this amount and usually was about 85–88 per cent. saturated. The following table shows the percentage saturation of the blood, withdrawn from the arteries of the persons indicated.

Saturation of Arterial Blood

	Subject	Altitude	Saturation	Pressure of O_2 in arterial blood	Pressure of O_2 in alveolar air
I	M.	Sea level	95 %	99 mm.	100 mm.[1]
		,,	95	100	101
		14,200 feet	83	—	—
		,,	91	58	56
	R.	Sea level	97	—	—
		14,200 feet	87·5	—	—
	B.	,,	84	—	—
	B'.	Sea level	95	—	—
		14,200 feet	82	—	—
II	McQ.	,,	86	57	59
	P.	,,	91	48	55
	McL.	,,	86	47	56
	C.	,,	87	55	54
III	Z.	,,	86	50	51
	V.	,,	82·5	50	—
	B.	,,	83·5	40	—

[1] See footnote page 68.

In the last two columns of the above table the pressures of oxygen in the alveolar air and in the arterial blood are given, for one of our party, for four engineers, and for one native. For two other natives the pressure in the arterial blood is given but not that in the alveolar air. It will be evident that the latter determination is one of great difficulty in the case of natives. Even in the case of hospital patients at home, alveolar air determinations by the method of Haldane and Priestly are extremely unreliable, because they demand a higher degree of education than persons unversed in exact methods possess; but the unreliability is enormously exaggerated in the case of persons who in addition are of low mentality and who speak a language which is not understood by the observer and which probably has to be interpreted through a third language, in which there are no terms corresponding to any scientific description of the routine. I mention this matter, not because I wish to excuse our only having obtained one reliable alveolar air determination on a native and not having brought home any determinations of vital capacity on them; both of these determinations we should have been glad to have. My object is rather to point out that there is a field, and I think there would be a welcome, for some one to go out to Cerro and settle down for long enough to train a number of the natives to give the sort of samples on which one could rely. It would need time, patience and perhaps a knowledge of their language, but I think it would be worth while. When we went to Cerro we were objects of the greatest suspicion to the natives. They understood that we wished for their blood—which in fact we did—though not in the sense which they understood the term. When we left we could have had a score of volunteers and probably as many more as we wished. This we owe largely to our American and British friends at Cerro.

I must return to the pressure of oxygen in the arterial blood. The direct measurements given above were obtained by transferring the blood, withdrawn into a 10 c.c. syringe by arterial puncture, to another syringe which contained enough mercury to fill the dead space and in addition a bubble of alveolar air so small that any change which took place between the blood and the air would not alter the composition of the former. The method was an obvious adaptation to human beings of that so brilliantly devised by Krogh [9] for rabbits, worked out with the help of Dr Nagahashi [10] who was working at Cambridge shortly before the expedition started for Peru.

The results show that the oxygen pressure in the arterial blood

was never sensibly above that in the alveolar air, the experimental
error being about 4 mm. In some cases it was a few millimetres
below that in alveolar air. The principal object achieved by the
determinations which I have just described is the definite proof that
the human body (and this is independent of all theories) can function
reasonably well when supplied with blood which may be as little as
82 per cent. saturated with oxygen. To have his oxygen saturation
cut down to this extent in the course of a short time is not likely
to be less inconvenient to a patient suffering from, say pneumonia,
than it is to a healthy person who goes up to the Andes, but 18 per
cent. of unsaturation, though it may be inconvenient and indeed
though it may give one a mild illness, is not likely, in itself, to be
fatal. Unsaturation is not the big factor of danger in pneumonia,
but it may be the rider which turns the scale. The value of oxygen
treatment, and there is abundant evidence that it has a value, is to
keep the patient going until the virulence of the toxine abates. This
in a percentage of cases it will do.

Having said the most important thing which emerged from the
data given in this chapter I would willingly close it, but it would be
unfair to my friend Dr Haldane, to whom I owe a great deal, not to
say a few more words about his theory. The form in which I have
stated it was as he held it at the time when I was most concerned
with it, that is to say in the early years of the war and at the time
when it was most attractive to me. In recent years he has altered it
and as I understand his position at present is as follows: The various
alveoli of the lung are ventilated to different extents, the majority
well, the minority ill, of these some secrete or may secrete. Therefore
blood containing oxygen at very different tensions A, B, C, D etc.,
and of different saturations W, X, Y, Z etc., emerging from different
parts of the lung gets mixed and so the blood which enters the
left heart, i.e. the arterial blood, possesses a saturation, M, which
is the mean of the saturations W, X, Y, Z, taking into account the
relative amounts of blood of each saturation. The resultant tension
will be the tension on the dissociation curve which corresponds to
the saturation M. This is something different from, and lower than
the T, the mean of the tensions A, B, C, D etc. Haldane's contention
is that T is the quantity measured by the carmine method, that if
M (which is the figure given in my table above) is equal to the tension
of oxygen in the alveolar air T will therefore be above it and the
secretion theory is proved. The term "arterial blood," as he uses it

now, does not connote "the blood in the arteries," as it obviously did in the quotation which I have given above from *Organism and Environment*, but the mathematical average of the bloods in the pulmonary venules.

This later adaptation to the secretory theory seems to me to have much less to commend it than had the theory ten years ago. It has lost as a theory, and it has lost in experimental support. Considered as a theory it has lost the attractive feature of achieving an object, that of supplying the tissues with blood which was approximately normal under conditions which would otherwise render it abnormal. From the experimental point of view the essence of the carmine method is that a certain partial pressure of CO, uniformly distributed over the lung is in equilibrium with the blood passing through the pulmonary capillaries. The later modification of his theory seems to deny even the possibility of this experimental basis, for if the CO pressure is uniform over the lung and the oxygen pressure varies in different alveoli, the blood will always be acquiring CO where the oxygen pressure is low and giving it out where the oxygen pressure is high. The assumed equilibrium will therefore never be attained.

BIBLIOGRAPHY

(1) HALDANE, J. S. *Journ. of Physiol.* XVIII. 201. 1895.

(2) BOHR, C. *Nagel's Handbuch*, I. 175. 1909.

(3) STADIE. *Journ. Exp. Med.* XXX. 215.

(4) HALDANE, J. S. *Organism and Environment as Illustrated by the Physiology of Breathing*, p. 56. Oxford, 1917.

(5) DOUGLAS, HALDANE, HENDERSON AND SCHNEIDER. *Phil. Trans.* B. CCIII. 185. 1912.

(6) See HALDANE, *Organism and Environment*. Oxford, 1917; *Mechanism, Life and Personality*. London, 1913.

(7) HILL, A. V. *Journ. of Physiol.* XLVI. p. xxvii. 1913.

(8) HALDANE, J. S. *Respiration*, 255. Yale Univ. Press. 1922.

(9) KROGH. *Skand. A. f. Physiol.* XX. 279. 1908.

(10) BARCROFT AND NAGAHASHI. *Journ. of Physiol.* LV. 339. 1921.

CHAPTER V

THE DIFFUSION OF OXYGEN THROUGH THE
PULMONARY EPITHELIUM

It is only fair to the secretion theory to institute some definite
enquiry whether the facts known regarding respiration can be explained by diffusion. This enquiry is very difficult because there are
certain significant facts which are not at our disposal. To these some
allusion will be made in due course. Nevertheless it is impossible
to shirk the whole subject.

One imagines that in the lung a large surface of capillaries is
exposed to the alveolar air. Mixed venous blood from the heart
enters into these capillaries and oxygen passes into the blood because
there is a higher pressure of oxygen in the alveolar air than in the
capillary blood. As the blood acquires oxygen the pressure of that
gas in it rises and diffusion takes place more and more slowly so
that as the blood passes along the vessel the pressure within it comes
more and more closely into equilibrium with that of the alveolar air.
It will be clear that the equilibrium can never be complete; that
could only take place if the capillary were of infinite length and if
the blood were to spend an infinite time going through it. One of
the items of knowledge which we would like is a statement of just
how nearly the equilibrium is struck.

We have then certain assumptions which it is not wise to take
for granted, but which for the moment we will accept. One is a
figure which we call the oxygen pressure in the alveolar air. This, for
purposes of calculation, we assume to be uniform over the lung,
and to be sufficiently uniform in an alveolus, that is to say at the
two ends of the same capillary, to give the phrase a meaning. The
other assumption which we have made and which I imagine to be
incorrect is that of a capillary surface of invariable area and invariable
average thickness. The third assumption which we are about to make
is that one can speak of an average oxygen pressure within the
capillary. Given these three assumptions, the known laws of diffusion
may be applied in this way. If P be the pressure of oxygen in the
alveolar air, p_1 be the average pressure of oxygen in the capillary
blood and Q the quantity of oxygen which diffuses from the alveolus
into the blood in a minute, then

$$Q = (P - p_1) \times K$$

where K is the constant, so long as the properties of the lung do not vary. If a particular case be selected in which $(P - p_1)$ was equal to 1, K would then equal Q. K, the diffusion coefficient, may then be defined as the quantity of oxygen which would diffuse through the lung per unit difference of pressure between the alveolar air and the capillary blood.

It is not easy to measure K directly for oxygen, but it is possible to measure it for carbon monoxide, and from the known properties of oxygen and carbon monoxide it may then be calculated for oxygen.

At high altitudes, of course, the difference of pressure between the oxygen in the alveolar air and that in the capillary is much reduced. It seemed extremely probable that at high altitudes the diffusion coefficient for oxygen would become larger, that is to say, the number of c.c. of oxygen which would go through the lung epithelium would increase for each millimetre difference of pressure. Such an increase would take place if the lung vessels dilated so far as to expose a larger surface of blood to the alveolar air. I say this seemed probable, perhaps I should give some reason for that faith, for at one time the possibility of dilatation of the vessels in the lung was denied on the basis of experiments performed by Brodie and Dixon [1]. But it is clear from the researches of Starling and Fühner [2] and of Mrs Tribe [3], (now Mrs Oppenheimer) that in the heart-lung preparation and even in the excised lung, dilatation of the vessels can be brought about with adrenaline. In the intact animal the question was gone into very thoroughly by Sir Edward Sharpey-Schafer [4], who showed beyond question that the vessels in the lung of the intact animal were under vaso-motor control.

Lastly, there are experiments by Dr John Shaw Dunn which always impressed me very much, possibly because I had the opportunity of seeing them. Dunn [5] measured the quantity of blood which passed through the lung per minute and the pressure in the right ventricle. These measurements were made with no other surgical operation than direct cardiac puncture passing the needle of a hypodermic syringe through the skin, chest wall, pericardium and heart wall into the cavity of the right or left ventricle as desired; the right ventricle for the measurement of the pressure, and both ventricles in order to obtain blood samples for the measurement of the blood flow, by the Porton method. Having found the values of the right intraventricular pressure and the minute-volume of blood passing through the chest, Dunn injected starch grains either into the jugular vein or into the right ventricle, sufficient in amount to cause a large proportion of the small arteries in the lungs to become embolised. The immediate result was a rise of pressure in the right ventricle which was transferred back into the jugular vein and a decrease in the minute-volume. These effects soon passed off and after ten minutes or so, bcth the right intraventricular pressure and the minute-volume had returned to their original values. It was not

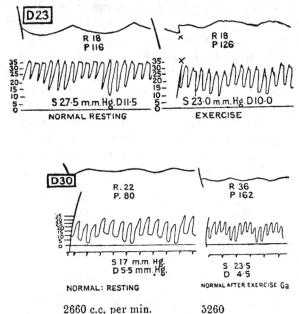

FIG. 20. Tracings of respiratory rhythm and normal right intraventricular pressure. R, respiration. P, pulse; vertical scale, pressure in centimetres of water. S, mean systolic and D, mean diastolic pressures expressed in mm. of Hg. Time, seconds.

that the emboli had been carried out of the pulmonary vessels by the blood stream, for post-mortem examination of the lung showed that the emboli were present in great abundance whilst the autopsies on other organs showed that no starch grains, or oil globules as the case might be, were to be found in the systemic circulation. He also showed that immediately active exercise caused by the goats running twice up and down a hill the mean pulmonary pressure was not raised. See Fig. 20.

	Systolic Pressure			Diastolic Pressure		
	Mean	Max.	Min.	Mean	Max.	Min.
Normal (1)	9·5	13·0	7·0	2·5	6·0	0·0
(2)	11·0	12·5	8·5	3·5	6·0	1·5
Exercise	12·5	18·0	8·0	2·5	8·0	−4·0

B

5

The only construction which could reasonably be put on Dunn's experiments was that the vessels in the non-embolised areas had opened out and by doing so had provided a vascular bed which presented no more resistance than that of the original. If then the vascular bed of the lung is of variable size, it seemed not unreasonable to suppose that it might be increased to a considerable extent at high altitudes. The gain to the system would be that, at the low oxygen pressure prevalent at such heights, the oxygen would have more time to diffuse into blood if the minute-volume were not increased, or alternatively, if the minute-volume were increased, the oxygen exchange required of each cubic centimetre of blood would be reduced so that less oxygen need pass through the wall of any one capillary.

We therefore made measurements of the diffusion coefficient (by the method described by Professor and Mrs Krogh[6], expecting an increase in the size of the capillary bed and as a corollary a rise in the diffusion coefficient, but no such change took place.

The following table gives the values of the diffusion coefficients as we found them for the various members of our party, at Lima and at Cerro.

Harrop	25·3	25·4
Bock	27·1	31·8
Barcroft	—	36·0
Binger	34·2	38·3
Doggart	—	42·6
Redfield	38·8	42·9
Forbes	46·8	43·8
Meakins	—	45·6

The diffusion coefficients, measured before and after the ascent, for five members of the party showed no more than a trivial change in any case and this not always in the same direction.

Perhaps I may digress for a moment to point out an interesting fact about these diffusion coefficients, i.e. that there is a very large variation as between person and person. Before going up to Cerro only Harrop (who measured the coefficients) and myself knew the results obtained at Lima; our reason for this secrecy was that the party had quite emphatic views before they went to Cerro as to whether or not they were likely to be overcome. Harrop wished to see if those having high diffusion coefficients stood the altitude better than the others and as he did not wish any psychological element to enter into the question he kept his counsel at Lima. The event however showed that the ones least affected were certainly those whose diffusion coefficients were over 40 and in this connection we may note that all the mining engineers whom Harrop investigated at Cerro had diffusion coefficients of the same order as the higher values for members of our party. The one exception to this was Rogers, who had a still higher coefficient. He had, I believe, been a prominent runner at his University.

The engineers' coefficients were as follows:

Phillpotts	...	...	...	43·4
McLaughlin	...	...	...	44·9
Cuthbertson	...	...	...	44·7
Colley ...	...	...	...	41·5
Rogers	...	...	...	65·3

Rogers's diffusion coefficient was two-and-a-half times Harrop's, and Harrop is by no means a person of mean development.

After this digression I must return to the consideration of the difficulties which attend the diffusion coefficient. I had said that the first was that of knowing the degree of possible variation in any one person.

Let me pass to the closer consideration of the actual terms involved—"the pressure of oxygen in the alveolar air" and the "mean difference of pressure between that and the pressure of oxygen in the capillary blood." Have these terms any real meaning? One visualised the alveolar air as being a sample obtained in some particular way, but is the composition of this sample the same as that of the gas in contact with the capillary wall? or is it a mixture of gases from various parts of the sponge work of the lung all of which may be included in the name alveolus, but some of which are of a much more atreal character than others. The conception of the Haldane-Priestley sample as being alveolar air has been one of enormous use to physiology, and even if the method has been improved upon for certain purposes the value of the general conception remains. One must admit therefore that the "alveolar sample" has proved its value as a useful approximation and therefore it demands our respect as something of proven value. One must remember also certain frailties of the human mind. One sees an alveolus in a microscopic preparation, or in a picture such as that of Miller which is given on page 34 of *Respiration* by Dr Haldane, and one is rather apt to visualise the alveolus—I speak for myself—as belonging to that order of magnitude. In point of fact an alveolus is about ·07 mm. in diameter and its diameter is therefore about equal to the thickness of a leaf of the *Journal of Physiology*. The length of time which would be required for a molecule of oxygen to diffuse that distance would be infinitesimally small. Perhaps, of all authors, Dr Haldane is more alive than any other to the limitations of his own method in this respect, and the reader should peruse his treatment of the subject in the work to which I have alluded. In the meantime there appear to be greater difficulties ahead, therefore let us concede for the moment that the Haldane-Priestley sample is a sufficiently close approximation, at all events when the subject is at rest.

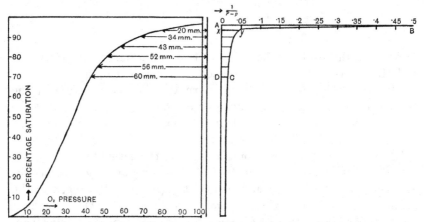

FIG. 21 a, in which the differences of pressure between the alveolar air and the blood is shown for given percentage saturations.

FIG. 21 b, in which the reciprocals of the same is shown for the given saturations.

The average difference of pressure between that of the oxygen in the blood and in the capillary is something much less tangible. It is a mathematical abstraction, the reader will understand what is meant only if he understands the conventional way of obtaining the quantity under consideration. I shall therefore describe it, taking a numerical example for the purpose.

Let me assume that A has an alveolar pressure of oxygen of 102 mm.; that his blood becomes saturated to within 2 mm.[1] of the alveolar pressure; that it therefore leaves the lung with a pressure of 100 mm. of oxygen; that the mixed venous blood arrives in the capillary of the lung with a saturation of 70 per cent. and therefore, according to the *intra vitam* dissociation curve of Christiansen, Douglas and Haldane (7), has a pressure of 42 mm. Having made these assumptions we proceed as follows:

[1] Work carried out by Bock whilst this book has been in the press places the difference at a much higher figure.

(1) Draw the *intra vitam* dissociation curves (Fig. 21 *a*).

(2) For suitable percentage saturations commencing with that of the arterial blood and ending with that of the venous blood read off the oxygen pressures thus:

A Percentage saturation	B Pressure (p) of O_2 mm.	C $P - p$ ($P = 102$ mm.)	D $\dfrac{1}{P - p}$	
96 %	100 mm.	2 mm.	·5	
94	82	20	·05	
90	68	34	·03	
85	59	43	·023	
80	50	52	·019	
75	46	56	·018	
70	42	60	·017	
94	**82**	**20**	**·05**	Mean by method of graphic integration

The pressures so obtained are subtracted from the pressure of oxygen in the alveolar air, 102 mm. giving the difference of pressure at each saturation between P, that in the alveolar air, and p, that in the arterial blood. The reciprocal of the pressure difference is then calculated, it will be found in column D. A graph, Fig. 21 *b*, is then drawn in which the percentage saturation is the ordinate and the value of $\dfrac{1}{P-p}$ is the abscissa. On this graph the value of $\dfrac{1}{P-p}$ is set off for each percentage saturation, the ends of the lines so drawn are joined and so an area A, B, C, D is obtained. This area is divided into two equal parts, by a horizontal line, xy. The principle of the method is that xy is the reciprocal of the mean difference of pressure (p_1) between the oxygen in the alveolar air and that in the capillary blood. In this case xy is approximately ·05, the mean value $\dfrac{1}{(P - p_1)}$ over the whole length of the capillary, ($P - p_1$) is therefore 20 mm. and since the alveolar pressure P is 102 mm., p_1 works out at 82 mm.

Suppose now the amount of oxygen being taken in by the person under these circumstances was 500 c.c. per minute the diffusion coefficient would be $\dfrac{500}{20} = 25$. That is the figure which Harrop found for himself.

A difficulty at once besets us. The area of the part above xy depends on the long spike which stretches out to ·5 (Fig. 21 *b*, AB). We have assumed that the difference between the final pressures of the arterial blood and alveolar air is 2 mm. So far as the possibility of measurements goes it might equally well be 0·2 mm., in which case the spike would be ten times as long and, though xy would only move upwards by a small fraction of 1 per cent. saturation, it would easily double in length, in which case the diffusion coefficient would be not 25 but 50. We may therefore lay down the principle that, if the diffusion coefficient is to be of the order which is obtained by Krogh's method of measurement, the pressure of oxygen in the blood which leaves the lung must not differ by more than about one milli- metre from that in the alveolar air. This relation we cannot measure with any certainty.

Another difficulty arises when an effort is made to calculate the maximum quantity of oxygen which the body can use. Suppose a person has a diffusion coefficient of 25, and suppose further he were taking in 3 litres of oxygen per minute which would probably be well within the competence of a person of Harrop's development, he would by calculation have an average difference of oxygen pressure of 120 mm., between his alveolar air and his capillary blood; which of course is impossible.

I gather from A. V. Hill that an athlete such as Rogers could absorb 4–6 litres of oxygen per minute, but for this performance even his diffusion coefficient of 65 could not avail him.

These I imagine are the sort of considerations which probably give more anxiety to Haldane than they do to some who criticise his theory. Evidently the diffusion theory requires some modifica- tion at this point, probably by giving much more consideration to the amount of blood passing through the lung and to area of the bed through which it passes. In either case one must suppose that the coefficient rises considerably when active exercise is taken.

And now to high altitudes. One man has a diffusion coefficient of 25, he is taking in 500 cubic centimetres of oxygen per minute, but the alveolar pressure is now 52 instead of 102. The average difference of pressure between his capillary blood and his alveolar air is to be the same as before, namely 20 mm. The average pressure in his blood must therefore be $52 - 20 = 32$ mm. According to the graph this will be found at 48 per cent. saturation. Calculate the arterial and venous saturations.

In a later chapter it will be shown that there is no great change in the blood flow and *ex hypothesi* the oxygen absorption is not altered, therefore the utilisation will be unaltered. Originally the arterial and venous saturations were 96 and 70 per cent. respectively, i.e. the utilisation was 26 per cent. and will still be 26 per cent. The problem is to mark out an area within the limits of the graph with the following properties: (a) the height must correspond to 26 per cent. of the ordinate, and (b) the portion of the area above 48 per cent. saturation shall have the same surface as that below. The upper limit *PQ* will be approximately at 60 per cent. saturation, the lower limit at 34 per cent. Here is something to make one consider. At rest the percentage saturation of the arterial blood was so close to what it would be if the alveolar air and the blood were shaken together *in vitro* that we could not tell the difference experimentally. But now a state of matters exists in which if the blood and the alveolar air were equilibrated the blood would be 81 per cent. saturated, whilst the highest saturation which it can attain under the circumstances assumed is 60 per cent. What does this signify? It means that while the capillary is long enough to admit of an approximate equilibrium being struck if the alveolar pressure is high, the capillary is too short (or the blood is too short a time in it) to make attainment of anything like an equilibrium possible when the oxygen pressure in the lung is halved.

Proceeding in this way one may calculate the percentage saturation of the oxygen in the arterial and mixed venous bloods, if the oxygen intake be increased or decreased, while the degree of utilisation, the alveolar O_2, and the diffusion coefficient be kept constant.

O_2 utilisation			26 %			
Diffusion coefficient			25			
O_2 pressure in alveolar air		102 mm.			52 mm.	
c.c. of O_2 absorbed per min.	250	500	750	250	500	750
Saturation in arterial blood	96 %	96 %	96 %	77 %	54 %	33 %
Saturation in venous blood	70	70	70	51	28	7

In the above table several things are particularly to be noted. Firstly, that at low altitudes a considerable variation may take place in the oxygen consumption without any sensible variation in the composition of the arterial or venous blood, given a constant degree of utilisation. A constant utilisation means that the minute-volume increases *pari passu* with the oxygen consumption. The reason of this constancy is because *xy* falls on the boundary of the spike and therefore can lengthen and shorten without moving appreciably up or down.

The second point to notice is that at any given consumption of oxygen the equilibrium is more nearly attained when the alveolar pressure is high than when it is low.

Thirdly, a relatively small increase in the oxygen consumption produces a great drop in the oxygenation of the arterial blood at low oxygen pressures. Thus while the arterial blood could conceivably achieve 81–82 per cent. saturation if left long enough in contact with the alveolar air at 52 mm. oxygen pressure, by the calculation with a diffusion coefficient of 25 it would only attain to 77 per cent. saturation if 250 c.c. of O_2 per minute were being taken in, 54 per cent. if 500 c.c. per minute were being taken in, and of 33 per cent. for an absorption of 750 c.c. of oxygen per minute.

In spite of all the difficulties which surround the diffusion theory there is this to be said in its favour—phenomena of the type which it requires do really occur in the following particulars:

(1) So far as our observations went the oxygen pressure determinations at sea-level showed no appreciable deficit in the saturation of the arterial blood, below that which it could acquire after a longer exposure to the alveolar air.

(2) A limited amount of exercise in animals makes very little difference to the saturation of the arterial blood. This I have not tested on man but I have frequently done so on animals[8], e.g.

		Oxygen saturation of arterial blood	
Rabbit	At rest	During muscular activity	After muscular activity
(1)	94 %	96 %	93 %
(2)	94	95	

Harrop[9] however has done experiments on man and informs me that he does not think there is satisfactory evidence of considerable want of saturation on moderate exercise.

(3) There was at Cerro a general tendency for just an appreciable gap to appear between the alveolar air oxygen pressures and those in the arterial blood. The average measurement in six cases amounted to 2–3 mm.

(4) There is a very common tendency to become cyanosed on exercise at high altitudes in a way which does not normally take place at the sea-level, and further measurements made on Meakins's blood showed that the percentage saturation of the arterial blood did drop at Cerro from 91 to 76 per cent. when exercise was taken, this drop was accompanied by great cyanosis. The cyanosis was only in part due to the fall in tension of the oxygen saturation in the arterial blood, the utilisation was increased, hence there was a double cause for the fall in saturation of the venous blood which occurred.

According to the diffusion theory an abnormal drop in the saturation of the arterial blood should appear not only when the subject is exposed to a low barometric pressure, but also at ordinary levels if the diffusion coefficient is greatly reduced. It is therefore of interest to compare the phenomenon presented by Meakins's blood at Cerro with similar states observed in rabbits and goats which have been so severely gassed as to render large portions of the lung useless on account of hepatisation and markedly to decrease the permeability of the rest.

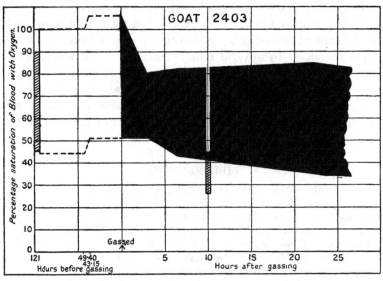

Fig. 22.

The following are observations on two such rabbits, which may be contrasted with the ungassed controls[8] the data of which were given above:

	Saturation of arterial blood	
Rabbit	At rest	During and after muscular activity
(3)	93 %	83, 80, 84 %
(4)	93	85, 87, 92

The above figure[10] shows the same phenomenon in a more marked way in a goat—the black area represents the utilisation, the top of the area therefore represents the oxygen saturation in the arterial blood, the bottom that in the venous blood. The general arterial saturation is markedly low and during exercise corresponding to an increased oxygen consumption of from 50 to 500 c.c. per kilo per hour the saturation of the arterial blood sinks from 82 to 45 per cent. and that of the venous blood correspondingly.

Finally, the reader may criticise the diffusion theory on the ground that it demands too much, that while the observations which we made agreed in sense with the demands of the theory they fell far short in degree. It would be so no doubt if the organism had not become in some ways acclimatised so as to broaden the basis on which the burden of anoxæmia is carried. A single instance may be mentioned here. The dissociation curve at Cerro is not the same as the one shown in Fig. 21 a, it is moved markedly to the left, so that at any saturation the difference of pressure between the alveolar air and the arterial blood is increased by several millimetres. So far as the saturation of the blood is concerned the effect is much the same as that of adding the same number of millimetres to the alveolar pressure. So far as the tissues are concerned it is otherwise, but the general effect of the shift in the curve is to spread what otherwise would be borne by the blood, jointly over the blood and the tissues.

BIBLIOGRAPHY

(1) Brodie and Dixon. *Journ. Physiol.* xxx. 476. 1904.
(2) Starling and Fühner. *Journ. Physiol.* xlvii. 286. 1913.
(3) Tribe, E. M. *Journ. Physiol.* xlviii. 154. 1914.
(4) Sharpey Schafer. *Quart. Journ. Exp. Physiol.* xii. 393. 1920.
(5) Dunn, J. S. *Quarterly Journ. Med.* xiii. 51, 131. 1919.
(6) Krogh, A. and M. *Skand. Arch.* xxiii. 236. 1910.
Krogh, M. *Journ. Physiol.* xlix. 271. 1915.
(7) Christiansen, Douglas and Haldane. *Journ. Physiol.* xlviii. 262. 1914.
(8) *Report* 14 *of the Chemical Warfare Medical Committee*, p. 19. 1918.
(9) Harrop. *Journ. Exp. Med.* xxx. 246. 1919.
(10) Barcroft. *Journal of the Royal Army Medical Corps.* January 1921. p. 6.

CHAPTER VI

MUSCULAR EXERCISE

Exertion is a predisposing cause to the whole train of symptoms which constitute mountain sickness. On the ascent of Monte Rosa from Alagna there are said to be three situations at which vomiting is likely to occur, the lowest of which is about 1000 feet below the laboratory at Col d'Olen, and therefore at an altitude of about 9000 feet. These three places are those at which, either by reason of the gradient or because of the force of the wind, the exertion of the climb is greater than elsewhere. If then muscular exercise will precipitate mountain sickness it is reasonable to commence an examination of the effects of rarity of the atmosphere by a consideration of the possible effects of oxygen want upon the process of muscular contraction.

Our ignorance of the effect of altitude on muscular contraction seems to be a little surprising when we recollect the ease with which exercise precipitates mountain sickness. The reason is probably not far to seek, the actual seat of the trouble is in the brain. The various symptoms are the direct effects of lack of oxygen supply to that organ. Muscular exercise accentuates the trouble because in one way or another, the activity of the muscles tends further to deprive the brain of oxygen; the organism therefore breaks down before the deleterious effect of oxygen want on the muscles becomes so apparent as itself to constitute a menace.

This is not to say that the conditions which obtain above 10,000 feet are without effect on the process of contraction in the human body, let us then jot down such information as is forthcoming in the hope that the points at issue may be taken up one by one by future workers, and that one day systematic work may be done on the subject. I say "jot down" rather than "put together" because to make any sort of story from such unsatisfactory material would be quite unwarrantable.

The basis of modern work on the processes essential to muscular contraction is that laid down in the work of Hopkins, Fletcher, Hill and their various collaborators. The gist of it so far as we are concerned is contained in two statements.

(1) That given an insufficient oxygen lactic acid appears as a

final product rather than as an intermediate product of muscular contraction.

(2) The lactic acid so formed may be oxidised by subsequent contact with sufficient oxygen.

What evidence is there of increased lactic acid formation at high altitudes?

Subject	Condition	Normal	Col d'Olen
Ryffel	Sleep	1	1·2
	Normal daily activity	2	—
Ryffel	Four hours' period, which included three hours' climbing, 7000 to 10,000 feet	—	3
Ryffel	Six hours, including four hours' climbing, 13,500 to 15,000 feet	—	2·2
Mathison	Four hours, including climb from 9000 to 10,000 feet in 19 minutes	—	2·7

First, let us consider the resting condition. The normal amounts of lactic acid put out in the urine during sleep and during ordinary daily activity may be taken as 1 and 2 milligrams per hour respectively. These may be compared with the results actually obtained at high altitudes (1).

The figures in the above table do not suggest any very striking increase in the elimination of lactic acid at altitudes up to 15,000 feet in the resting organism, or in slightly active organism, as the result of oxygen want. Certainly the increased elimination of lactic acid seems to be in no way commensurate with the distress which is experienced. There is however the possibility of increased lactic acid production by the muscles and of its subsequent combustion in the body.

Let us therefore turn to the percentage of lactic acid found in the blood—a subject on which we possess more complete data. The following table shows the results of determinations carried out by Ryffel's (2) method. It cannot be claimed that Ryffel's method commands as much confidence as some of the more modern ones, nevertheless the results when tabulated appear worthy of respect so far as they go. The duplicates on the same person at different sea-level stations and different times seem fairly consistent. The table shows pretty clearly that up to 10,000 feet there is no excess of lactic acid in the blood. There are but two determinations at 15,000 feet and these show approximately a three-fold increase in the lactic acid in the blood. It should be added that the blood taken at the Capanna Margherita hut was shed the morning after our arrival there. There is no information as to whether the excessive lactic acid in the blood which was then found would have been maintained.

The excess of lactic acid amounted to about 25 mg. per 100 c.c. of blood, or taken over the whole five litres of circulating fluid it would "tot up" to something over one gram.

What happens to this gram of lactic acid? Here is another question which might be worth following up. It will not have escaped the reader that, at the rate at which the acid is leaving the body in the urine, 500 to 1000 hours would be required for its elimination. Perhaps it is oxidised in the body. This seems very likely to be the case in general principles and evidence which could be used in favour of such a view will be given later.

Percentage of Lactic Acid in Blood

| Name | Approximate sea-level | | 10,000 feet | | 15,000 feet | |
	Place		Col d'Olen	Gain on Pisa	Capanna Margherita	Gain on Pisa
Roberts	Pisa	·012	·018	+ ·006	·039	·027
Camis	Pisa	·013	·017	+ ·004	·036	·021
Ryffel	Pisa	·014	·018	+ ·004	—	—
Ryffel	London	·014	·019	+ ·005	—	—
Mathison	Pisa	·015	·013	− ·002	—	—
Barcroft	Pisa	·024	—	—	—	—
Barcroft	Carlingford	·021	—	—	—	—

If however this excess of lactic acid is oxidised in the body one is forced back to the question: Is its presence in the blood necessarily a sign of increased lactic acid production? It may be so, but I think it is *not* necessarily so. Consider the matter in the simplest possible light and suppose merely that you are dealing with a physico-chemical system which obeys the law of mass action. (1) Assume that the muscles are at the sea-level putting a certain amount of lactic acid into the blood which we shall call $X \pm 1$ mgs. per hour. (2) This lactic acid (with the exception of 1 mg. excretion per hour) is oxidised at such a rate as to maintain the concentration in the blood constant, that is to say X grams per hour are oxidised. (3) The rate of oxidation varies with the product of C_L (the concentration of lactic acid) and C_O (that of the concentration of oxygen) in the blood. From these assumptions it follows that if X mgs. of lactic acid are to be oxidised when the concentration of oxygen (C_O) in the blood is reduced it can only be done by increasing the concentration of the lactic (C_L) so that ($C_L \times C_O$) remains constant.

It may be argued that whereas at the Capanna Margherita the concentration of oxygen in the plasma of the arterial blood was still more than half that at the sea-level, the concentration of lactic acid increased three-fold, so that ($C_L \times C_O$) in the arterial blood was in point of fact greater at 15,000 feet than at the sea-level. This I mention merely to brush aside; neither the accuracy of the lactic acid estimation, nor the assumption that the "arterial blood" is "the blood," nor our knowledge of the system with which we have to do, warrant any such close argument from the data.

The important facts seem to be:

(1) The evidence so far as it goes points to increased lactic acid in the blood at 15,000 feet. Such effects, if any, as may be caused by a specific increase in the acid will follow.

(2) There is no certain evidence of lactic acid formation.

(3) The effects of lactic acid increase therefore "may," I do not say "do," take place at high altitudes without any actual increase in the formation of the same.

So much for the formation of lactic acid.

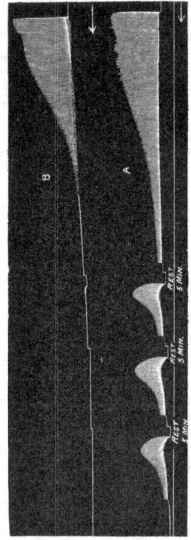

FIG. 23. (Fletcher.) Reads from right to left. Fatigue in a pair of Sartorii. Max. break shocks one per second. Load 6 grams. Temp. 19° C. A, exposed to oxygen. B, exposed to nitrogen.

Among the many instructive experiments by which Fletcher (3) demonstrated the relation between oxygen want and fatigue in excised frog's muscle, the figure on p. 78 records the one which I have always singled out to show my class.

The tracings A and B are those of two gastrocnemius muscles taken from the same frog. They are made at each twitch to lift equal weights, the difference between them is that A is in an atmosphere of oxygen, B is in an atmosphere of nitrogen. The interpretation of these two tracings, in the light of the researches of which they form a part, is as follows: In the case of each muscle there was some degree of fatigue, in B it was complete in about three minutes, in A it was considerable but not complete at the end of five minutes.

Shocks of uniform strength and frequency were passing into the muscle up to this point. The completely fatigued muscle B ceased to contract in response to the shocks after three minutes, the incompletely fatigued muscle A, still responded at the end of five minutes but with contractions much reduced in height. The cause of the fatigue was the accumulation of lactic acid in the muscles in the vessels of which no circulation was taking place. The reason of the lactic acid accumulation in each muscle was that in the process of contraction that material was being manufactured more rapidly than it was being oxidised. In muscle B however this disproportion was much greater than in muscle A, for in muscle B none of the lactic acid was being oxidised, there being no available oxygen, whilst in muscle A a certain proportion was being oxidised by such oxygen as was able to diffuse from the atmosphere through the tissue of the muscle. No doubt the outer fibres were relatively unfatigued whilst those in the heart of the muscle were fatigued. Accepting this explanation let us pass to the part of the tracing which is of most interest in the present connection, namely, the effect of giving each muscle five minutes rest. In muscle B the rest does not reduce the fatigue—in a sense it is improperly called rest—but in A the fatigue is very much lessened because the lactic acid is capable of being oxidised in the muscle itself after it is formed for a period of time which amounts at least to minutes. The material point then is that the lactic acid which is formed as the result of contraction in deficient oxygen supply can be oxidised in the muscle a long time (as compared with the time taken by a contraction) after it is formed.

Now let us pass to consider some observations on the oxidation in mammalian muscle in the light of what has just been said.

Verzàr[4], on the gastrocnemius of the intact cat made a long series of experiments in which he estimated the oxygen used by the muscle before, during, and after tetanisation. His results fell into two categories:

(1) Those in which the oxygen used during tetanisation was at a less rate than during rest.

(2) Those in which it was used at a greater rate than during rest.

In both cases there was an excessive oxygen consumption after the tetanus, so that in all cases the rate of oxygen consumption at some moment after the tetanus was greater than during the tetanus, and the sum of the oxygen used after the tetanus and that used during the tetanus was greater than would have been used in an equal period of rest.

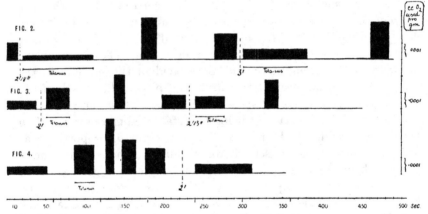

Fig. 24. Oxygen used by gastrocnemius of muscle. Ordinate c.c. per gram. Abscissa = seconds. The dotted vertical lines signify points at which the drum was stopped.

The only explanation of these results which seemed likely was that the muscles were in some degree asphyxiated. The only plausible explanation of a fall in oxygen consumption of a muscle during tetanus as compared with rest, was that the blood supply of the muscle was interfered with and that its oxygen supply was impaired. As regards the increased oxygen consumption after the contraction was over, or as Hill and Lupton[5] now call it "the oxygen debt," it is clear from the work of Fletcher and Hopkins that this "debt" represents the oxygen used in oxidising lactic acid formed by the partially asphyxiated muscle.

It did not seem possible to leave the matter at this point, so when the opportunity served Toyojiro Kato(6) and I repeated Verzàr's experiments but with such modifications as insured a better blood supply to the muscle. The experiments, five in number, were done on the dog. Three were on the gastrocnemius and two on the digastric.

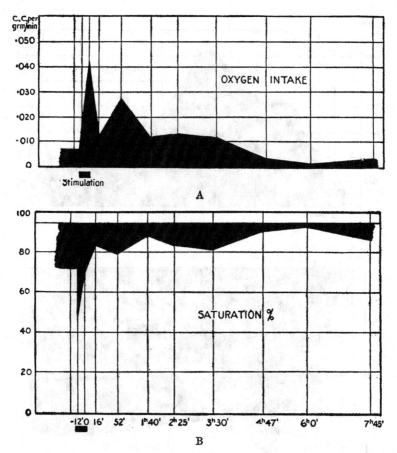

FIG. 25. A, oxygen intake of muscle with abundant blood flow. B, percentage saturation of blood with oxygen, the top of the black area representing the percentage saturation of the arterial blood and the bottom the venous blood. Abscissa = time from end of stimulus.   Signal = period of stimulation.

The stimulus took the form not of one continuous tetanus but over a period of 15 minutes stimuli were given during 0·3 of each second. Of the five experiments four differed from those of Verzàr by showing a much larger consumption during the exercise than during the previous period of rest, or the subsequent period of recovery, thus our conjecture that the delay in oxidation due to deficient oxygen supply seemed to be correct, and indeed it was confirmed by the fifth experiment which gave a result similar to those of Verzàr's in which the oxygen consumption increased during exercise but attained

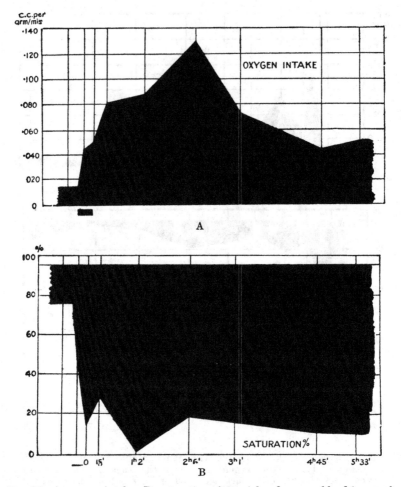

Fig. 26. A, oxygen intake. B, saturation of arterial and venous blood in muscle ill-supplied with blood, data figured as in Fig. 25.

its maximum after cessation of the exercise. The reason why I say that the fifth experiment confirmed our conjecture is that in it the muscle was known to be functioning with a very restricted supply of oxygen; the details of this experiment seem so important that they may be compared in some detail with those of one in which the oxygen supply was much more ample.

The point at issue may be grasped from the comparison of Fig. 25 with Fig. 26. The black signal underneath the base-line marks time during which the muscle was made to contract. In Fig. 25, A, the oxygen consumption rises to its maximum—about six times the resting value—during the stimulation, falls suddenly afterwards and for some hours shows indications of oxygen debt, but only on one occasion after the tetanus ceased was the oxygen consumption greater than twice that before the stimulation. Without laying too much stress on the one determination 52 minutes from zero, we may say that in the intact muscle under experimental conditions but with good blood supply, there is a considerable amount of material left in the muscle which is there oxidised after the contraction is over, but that the rate at which this oxidation takes place is much less than during the contractions. In Fig. 26, as will be seen from the portion marked B, the blood leaving the muscle was almost completely reduced for five hours after the tetanus, the blood flow being very slow throughout. The most intense oxidation was after and not during the exercise.

Let us pass from such muscles as that referred to in Figs. 25 and 26 where a muscle, which though in the body and supplied with blood from the heart, has been dissected free from other tissue, has been cooled at its surface and has no doubt suffered in other ways, to those which are doing their work in the normal process of bodily exercise. It is not possible to isolate the oxygen used by these muscles from that used up by the whole body.

The experiments of Douglas and Campbell (7), Lupton and Long (8), and Krogh and Lindhard (9) all agree in showing: (1) that during muscular work there is a great increase in the oxygen consumption of the body; (2) that the oxygen consumption does not fall for some time after the cessation of the exercise to the pre-exercise figure; (3) that even after hard exercise in ordinary atmospheric air the oxygen debt of the body is trifling as compared with that shown in Fig. 25, and is therefore much farther removed from that shown in Fig. 26.

Nevertheless, after severe exercise the body does accumulate an oxygen debt so that the difference between the body as a whole and that of the muscles described is one of degree and not of kind. The debt as shown in Fig. 27 is greater and takes much longer to pay off when the exercise is taken in an atmosphere of only 14 per cent.

oxygen than when taken in air. The difference in degree is however sufficient to demand some explanation:

(1) It must be admitted quite freely that any muscle nerve preparation in the living animal is, so far as our experience has carried us, very far from being an ideal preparation. In order to be able to collect the blood which comes from the muscle and from that only, the whole gastrocnemius must be dissected out, all the collateral

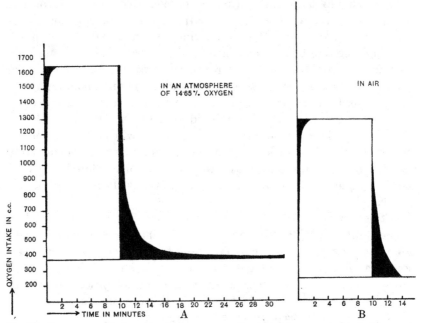

Fig. 27. Oxygen used in ten minutes' severe exercise which is purported to be the same in quantity in A and B. The white area represents the oxygen absorbed during the exercise, the black area following it the oxygen debt. A, exercise taken in 14·65 per cent. oxygen. B, exercise taken in air. Note the oxygen debt is more protracted in A than in B[1].

vessels (some of which are in the most inaccessible places adjacent to the knee-joint and deep to the muscle) must be tied, and in general the tissue must be man-handled to a degree which cannot but leave its functional activity considerably impaired. So far then the comparison goes entirely in favour of judging of the extent of oxygen debt from the metabolism of the body as a whole, and accepting the much lower estimates which that method yields.

(2) There is this difference between Kato's and my experiments and those of workers on the body, namely, that the muscles on which we

[1] Work from A. H. Hill's Laboratory carried out while this has been in press throws doubt on the degree of oxygen debt shown in Fig. 27, A.

experimented were fatigued to a standstill. The reason may have been due partly to the unsatisfactory conditions which enabled an unduly small amount of contraction to fatigue the fibre completely. It is not so much the reason as the fact which we are emphasising at the moment. I think it would be generally admitted that if the human body was exercised till the muscle fibres lost or nearly lost their contractility the oxygen debt would be much greater than it is.

(3) Lastly, there is one small point in favour of the intact muscle nerve preparation as compared with the body as a whole. In the muscle intact nerve preparation, the nerve of which has been cut for some hours, the "resting" condition is one in which the metabolism is reduced to its basal level. In the body the "pre-exercise" state of the muscles is one in which they are in a condition of tone—a condition in which Zuntz supposed about twice as much oxygen to be used as when the nerve was cut. Let us call the oxygen consumption of the muscle with the cut nerve 1, that of the resting muscle in the body 2, and that during the period of exercise 20. It may be that after severe exercise the muscle falls back to a condition in which such tone as is maintained involves a lower degree of metabolism than before the exercise and which therefore only demands an oxygen consumption of 1·5. Now if the oxygen used by the body is the same before and after the exercise, then a consumption of ·5 will be oxygen debt. Let me be quite clear in saying that I know of no positive facts one way or other as to the relative degrees of tone before and after the contraction; the point I do wish to emphasise is that in Kato's and my experiments there was no possibility of marking the payment of the oxygen debt by the establishment of economy in other regions, while in the experiments involving metabolism of the body as a whole that possibility exists.

Considering the whole series of observations starting with experiments on the excised frog's muscle (which in nitrogen has no oxygen supply), passing through experiments on the intact muscle nerve preparation (with oxygen supplied, perhaps not very efficiently by the blood stream) and ending with the muscle as it functions in the normal body, the following generalisations seem warranted. (1) In the excised muscle nerve preparation in nitrogen the whole metabolism is oxygen debt. (2) In the intact muscle nerve preparation the oxygen debt is always abnormally large and is even more excessive when the blood supply is restricted. (3) In the normal muscle the oxygen debt still exists if the exertion is great, but is relatively trifling. (4) In excised frog's muscle the oxygen debt is contracted by the formation of lactic acid in the muscle which must be oxidised if the muscle is to pass out of the fatigued condition. Presumably the same is true of the oxygen debt in the intact muscle nerve preparation and even in the whole animal. It is proven in the case of the frog but it remains to be proven in the case of the intact animal.

Let us picture to ourselves firstly the conditions as regards oxygen supply under which muscle normally contracts, and then let us consider how a modification of these conditions affects the actual process of contraction.

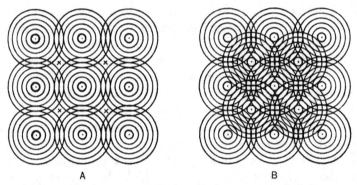

A   B

FIG. 28. A, area with nine open capillaries. Each concentric circle is supposed to represent a drop of 5 mm. oxygen pressure from that in the capillary which is 30 mm. The X's represent areas of no pressure. B, thirteen capillaries in the same area. Most of the tissue is supplied from more than one capillary. No areas of zero pressure.

Verzàr (10) showed that if the oxygen pressure in the arterial blood is appreciably cut down the gastrocnemius muscle (the nerve of which was cut) uses less oxygen than previously. The following interpretation of this fact was given by Krogh (11). Consider a cross-section of the muscle which we may suppose to consist schematically of parallel fibres fed with oxygen by capillaries which run parallel to them. Both the fibres and the capillaries are seen in the section cut perpendicularly. Of the capillaries a few are patent and through them runs blood, but the majority are shut and need not be considered in the first instance.

The oxygen is at a certain pressure p in the capillary from which it radiates out into the surrounding tissue by which it is being used so that the pressure gradually falls as the distance from the capillary increases. We may suppose that the pressure in the capillary is 30 mm. Round this we may draw contour lines which represent the oxygen pressures at the various situations round the capillaries. Just where the zones supplied by adjacent open capillaries meet the oxygen pressure is zero (such a point is marked × in Fig. 28), but the area in which this is the case is so small as to be negligible. Two facts stand out: (1) there is an area with zero oxygen pressure. (2) This area is minute enough to be hypothetical. The conjunction of these two facts depends upon the balance of three factors: (1) the quantity of oxygen being used by the muscle, (2) the number of open capillaries, (3) the pressure in each. If the quantity of oxygen used, and the capillary pressure remained constant and more capillaries opened, as in Fig. 28, B, there would be a positive oxygen pressure everywhere, whilst if fewer capillaries were open considerable areas would appear in which there was no oxygen pressure and in which therefore no oxidation could take place.

Or again, suppose the oxygen consumption and the number of open capillaries to remain constant: then if the oxygen pressure in each capillary is increased there will be a positive pressure everywhere, whilst if the tension of oxygen in the capillary drops anærobic areas will appear in the muscle. This evidently was the position of affairs in Verzàr's muscles. The oxygen pressure and the number of open capillaries were so nicely adjusted to the needs of the muscle, that any cutting down of the capillary oxygen pressure opened out considerable areas of muscle to which no oxygen penetrated and therefore the oxygen used by the whole muscle was reduced.

So great are the possibilities of increased capillary supply, as is evident from the calculations of Krogh, that actual asphyxiation of the muscle substance is not a very serious factor in ordinary exercise at high altitudes, and therefore the effects of the altitude must for the most part be sought elsewhere.

BIBLIOGRAPHY

(1) BARCROFT, CAMIS, MATHISON, ROBERTS AND RYFFEL. *Phil. Trans. Roy. Soc.* B. CCVI. 49. 1914.

(2) RYFFEL. *Proc. Physiol. Soc., Journ. Physiol.* XXXIX. p. ix. 1909.

(3) FLETCHER, W. M. *Journ. Physiol.* XXVIII. 492. 1902.

(4) VERZÀR. *Journ. Physiol.* XLIII. 243. 1912.

(5) HILL AND LUPTON. *Physiol. Proc., Journ. Physiol.* LVI. p. xxxii. 1922.

(6) BARCROFT AND KATO. *Phil. Trans. Roy. Soc.* B. CCVII. 149. 1915.

(7) CAMPBELL, DOUGLAS AND HOBSON. *Ibid.* CCX. 1. 1920.

(8) LUPTON AND LONG. Unpublished.

(9) KROGH AND LINDHARD. *Journ. Physiol.* LIII. 431. 1920.

(10) VERZÀR, F. *Journ. Physiol.* XLV. 39. 1912.

(11) KROGH, A. *Journ. Physiol.* LII. 457. 1919.

CHAPTER VII

THE HYDROGEN-ION CONCENTRATION
OF THE BLOOD

AFTER this somewhat lengthy digression let me return to the subject of mountain sickness. I had mentioned that the symptoms were attributed by Paul Bert[1] to an actual want of sufficient molecules of oxygen in each cubic foot of air inspired into the lungs. This view of the matter was not allowed to go unchallenged for long. Mosso, who, as I have said, was the great moving force in the study of high altitudes, put forward a rival theory, based on the fact that the expired air contained less carbonic acid at high altitudes than at the sea-level. Workers who have followed him have verified the facts, and expanded them so as to include the alveolar air. Sooner or later, sometimes sooner, sometimes later, every one who goes up high enough gets a diminution of carbonic acid in the expired air, in the alveolar air, and in the blood. This condition was called by Mosso[2] "acapnia" and to it he attributed the effects of mountain sickness. The condition of acapnia has become increasingly important within the last decade or so, not because of its possible relation to mountain sickness, but because of the work of Professor Yandell Henderson[3] at Yale, who, of course, has investigated the condition very thoroughly, especially in its bearing on surgical shock. In some very important respects Henderson's work has received striking confirmation at the hands of Dale quite recently.

I should like to make Mosso's view of the ætiology of acapnia quite clear, but my difficulty in doing this is the fact that I have never quite been able to grasp it myself. Henderson in his work on the subject started from an intelligible point of view, namely, that during, say, an abdominal operation the forced respiration of the subject causes a considerable dissipation of carbonic acid which would not otherwise have taken place. If therefore the body be producing carbonic acid at a uniform or reduced rate and expelling it at an increased rate the quantity held by the blood and tissues must drop. Mosso however had no such intelligible ground on which to base his acapnia theory of mountain sickness. He supposed that mere reduction of barometric pressure would of itself extract the carbonic acid from the body—much as a soda-water bottle would yield its CO_2 if the cork were taken out. I speak with all deference, but Mosso seems to me to have overlooked the fact that the body is exposed to what is practically a vacuum of CO_2, whether it be at the Capanna Margherita or in his own laboratory at Turin.

The position then at the end of Mosso's life may be briefly stated in the following table:

SCHEME 1

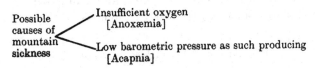

Possible causes of mountain sickness

Insufficient oxygen [Anoxæmia]

Low barometric pressure as such producing [Acapnia]

Granting the possibility of the existence of acapnia, the further question would arise: How does the acapnia produce its supposed results? There are two possible ways in which it might be held to act. The first is that the absence of CO_2 *per se* should affect the functions of the body, the second is that other things being equal the evaporation of CO_2 from the blood would render that fluid more alkaline. This alkalinity would be reflected by the tissues generally and might affect their function.

The table which I have given above as expressing the causes of mountain sickness then might be expanded as follows and the alternatives then would be:

SCHEME 2

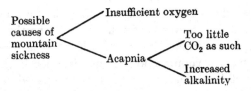

Possible causes of mountain sickness

Insufficient oxygen

Acapnia

Too little CO_2 as such

Increased alkalinity

Such then was the position when the subject became one of first hand interest to me. In 1909 the late Professor Zuntz of Berlin sent me a very pleasant invitation. It contained the news that he was about to organise an expedition to Teneriffe the following year. This expedition was to be international in character and he asked me to accompany him and to bring another English worker with me. I was fortunate in having Dr Douglas as my colleague. The results which we brought back from Teneriffe shed some light on each of the possible mechanisms of acapnia. Let us first consider whether or not the mere reduction of CO_2, as such, in the blood is responsible for mountain sickness.

There was one member of the party who never showed any degree of acapnia at any time in Teneriffe—that unfortunately was myself. I say unfortunately because I was the only worker who was at all incapacitated by the air at the Alta Vista Hut. The following table shows partial pressure of carbonic acid in my blood at various altitudes and also of Dr Douglas. He was perfectly free from all symptoms, as also were Professors Zuntz and Durig whose CO_2 ran somewhat similar courses to that of Dr Douglas(4).

Pressure of CO_2 *in alveolar air mm.*

			Sea Level Europe	Cañadas	Alta Vista
Douglas	...	...	41	36	32
Barcroft	...	...	40	41	38
Zuntz ...	...	...	35	29	27

The above table shows that as between the sea-level and the Alta Vista Hut, there was a drop of more than 20 per cent. in the alveolar CO_2 tensions of Zuntz and Douglas. There was no such drop in my case. The drop of 7 or 9 mm. in the alveolar CO_2 is caused of course by increased total ventilation on their parts, as a corollary to which there was a corresponding rise in alveolar oxygen. Zuntz and Douglas have alveolar oxygen pressures of some ten millimetres above my own. Now if reduced CO_2 pressure were the cause of mountain sickness Zuntz and Douglas should have been the sufferers, if reduced oxygen pressure in the alveolar air were the cause I would be the victim, as, in fact, I was to some extent. This experiment was controlled on Monte Rosa where my carbonic acid pressure dropped in the ordinary way and where I did not suffer at all. I am prepared therefore to delete "reduction of CO_2 as such" from the scheme of possible causes of mountain sickness which now stands as follows:

SCHEME 3

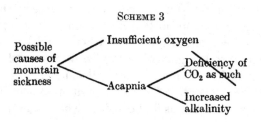

Let us now turn to another possibility which the acapnia theory presents, namely that of decreased alkalinity of the blood. On our return from Teneriffe I was quite of the opinion that it might be deleted as well. The argument was as follows. The affinity of hæmoglobin for oxygen depends upon the circumstances under which the hæmoglobin is placed, it decreases with a rise of temperature, with a rise in hydrogen-ion concentration, and it is also influenced by salts. Small additions of salt to blood do not however produce any appreciable effect on the affinity of the hæmoglobin for oxygen. On the other hand, small changes in hydrogen-ion concentration do produce a very marked effect. At constant temperature then my idea was that if the alkalinity of the blood increased the hæmoglobin would gain in its affinity for oxygen to an extent which might be discernible. This matter was tested on the bloods of each member of the party. As the result of these tests it appeared that when the blood, drawn at any given altitude, was exposed to any standard pressure of oxygen, in the presence of the concentration of carbonic acid which the actual blood contained in the body at that altitude. Scheme 3 then turned into Scheme 4.

SCHEME 4

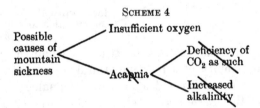

The method which I used, like all indirect methods, has certain weaknesses. Of these the principal one is the assumption that the reaction inside the red corpuscle is an index of the reaction of the plasma. The whole by-play between the corpuscles and the plasma was undiscovered at that time. This point I must take up in detail later. Here I merely wish to emphasise the point that any modern work on the subject would be considered unsatisfactory that did not directly measure the hydrogen-ion concentration of the plasma itself. Though our conclusion was confirmed by Hasselbalch and Lindhard in a chamber test using the platinum electrode to measure the CH of the blood, it was one of our objects in going to Peru, but we had more reasons for doing so than that of adding one more nail to the coffin of the acapnia theory. The reaction of the blood has a very direct bearing upon the rival theory, that of supposing the medullary centres to be upset by oxygen want, or, as the phrase goes, anoxæmia.

I have pointed out that in Teneriffe the oxygen pressure in my alveolar air was perhaps ten millimetres below that in the air cells of Dr Douglas or Professor Zuntz.

Granting therefore that mountain sickness is in some way or other to be referred to a too low partial pressure of oxygen in the lungs, one must probe the possible mechanisms by which anoxæmia can produce its effect. These bear a strange similarity to the investigations which we have already studied with regard to carbonic acid. Of two possible alternative mechanisms the one depends upon the hydrogen-ion concentration of the blood and the other on the specific effects of the gas—or rather of its absence. The latter view is not free from a certain intellectual difficulty. To say that "you are made to vomit by the oxygen which is not there" would be to reveal my nationality, but if I put the matter just in that way you will appreciate a side of the question which many minds do not find easy to grasp. We therefore arrive at the following scheme:

SCHEME 5

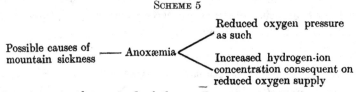

Let us turn to the second of these. It at least had the advantage of offering the possibility of a positive stimulus and not a negative one; further there was a good deal, by way of analogy, to make it likely. Haldane and Priestley [5] believed that the breathlessness of exercise was due to increased CO_2 in the blood. That the CO_2 as such was not the cause is shown by the fact that after severe exercise, the breathlessness is maintained in spite of the fact that the concentration of CO_2 in the blood becomes abnormally low. The factor common to both conditions is the increase in the hydrogen-ion concentration. Lewis, Cotton, Ryffel, Wolf and I [6] had put forward the view, which has since in the main been confirmed by Fraser, Ross and Dreyer [7] using more up-to-date methods, that the dyspnœa in certain types of cardiac trouble was associated with and probably due to increased hydrogen-ion concentration of the blood.

The actual evidence of increased hydrogen-ion concentration in the plasma of the *resting* body at high altitudes was unsatisfactory. It is very necessary to separate in one's mind the conditions of rest and exercise. There was good reason to suppose that the acid production to which exercise gives rise took place on a larger scale at high altitudes than at low ones as was shown in the preceding chapter (8). Here however we are dealing solely with the resting condition of the body, and, as we said, the evidence of increased hydrogen-ion concentration at rest was very unsatisfactory. There was plenty of evidence that the hydrogen-ion concentration of the CO_2 free blood increased as the altitude rose, but likewise the CO_2 concentration decreased, and the question then was whether the decrease of CO_2 was, or was not, counterbalanced by the decrease of alkali in the plasma.

In 1910 Yandell Henderson (9), and later Henderson and Haggard (10), performed a series of observations which tended strongly to divert opinion in the direction of oxygen want as such being the cause of the breathlessness at high altitudes. Submitting dogs to a deficiency of oxygen, they showed that the following was the order of events, first, the dyspnœa, secondly, the loss of CO_2 by the blood as the effect of the over ventilation, thirdly, the increased *hydroxyl*-ion concentration of the blood, and fourthly, the restoration of the blood reaction owing to secretion of alkali by the kidney. This, which is sometimes called the "alkalosis" as opposed to the acidosis theory, was strongly supported by Haldane, who with Kellas and Kennaway (11), using a chamber filled with rarefied air, showed that the same secretion of alkali in the urine took place in men, as Henderson and Haggard had found in dogs.

A direct test of the hydrogen-ion concentration of the plasma of blood equilibrated with the CO_2 pressure, proper to the place and person, had never been made at high altitudes, though Hasselbalch and Lindhard (12) had carried it out in a chamber and found an increased hydrogen-ion concentration, though one within the limits of experimental error. These observations were carried out at a barometric pressure of 589 mm. which corresponds to about 7000 feet—too low an altitude to be decisive. Sundstrœm found a slight acidæmia by indicators. It was part of our programme to try this test in Peru, and perhaps it was for the purpose of doing so more than for any other that we desired a thoroughly good laboratory.

The result of our labours were, I am sorry to say, far from being so complete as we could have desired. Perhaps the point which we proved most definitely was that a complete and satisfactory research could be carried out on the subject at Cerro by our successors if they were prepared to take as many weeks as we had taken days. Nevertheless, we did not come back quite empty-handed. Three methods of testing the hydrogen-ion concentration of the plasma were attempted: (1) the Dale-Evans[13] method, (2) the electrometric, and (3) the ratio of the combined carbonic acid in the blood.

Of the electrometric method the only thing to be said is that it could be got to work, and if the glass electrode which has been elaborated by W. E. L. Brown[14] turns out to be a success for routine measurement, I hope Brown or, failing him, another, will take it to Cerro and repeat our determinations.

Concerning the Dale-Evans method, the following figure summarises the determinations made. The unsatisfactory point is that while the members of each group averaged were very close together the averages at different places at the sea-level for the same person are often a good way apart.

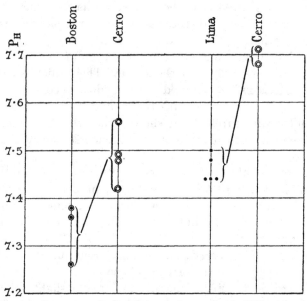

FIG. 29. Showing the extreme limits of change in reaction in Binger's and Redfield's blood respectively by the Dale-Evans method. The actual change may be anything between *nil* and the result shown.

A point in the figure is probably the average of four such determinations as 7·53, 7·56, 7·50, 7·53; mean 7·54. The determinations by the CO_2 method were much more numerous. They are shown in Fig. 30.

The one thing which I think one can say from these figures is that they give no support to the idea that the blood is more acid at high altitudes than at low ones. For the rest they are conflicting. It may be that the experimental error is so large as to make the decision impossible as to whether the blood is of the same hydrogen-ion concentration or is more alkaline, or it may be that the blood passes through a phase of greater alkalinity and settles down ultimately to that of the man as he was at the sea-level. This point we must leave for future workers. In either case I think no one would now say that the alkalinity of the blood, if it exists, was the cause and not the effect of the reaction of the organism to high altitude and unless some new factor appears I for one am prepared to subscribe to the general view for which Yandell Henderson and Haldane are the protagonists, namely, that the cause of dyspnœa at high altitudes is the direct and not the indirect effect of an insufficient supply of oxygen to the medulla, rendering the respiratory centre more irritable.

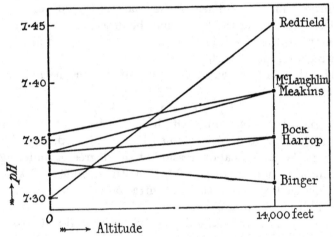

Fig. 30. Measured changes in hydrogen-ion concentration by the CO_2 method uncorrected for any change in the quantity of hæmoglobin present.

So much for rest. In the case of work our results quite bore out those obtained by the Monte Rosa expedition [8] of 1911, namely, that a less amount of work will produce a given change in the hydrogen-ion concentration of the blood at high altitudes than at low ones, as the following figures show, a result which agrees with that obtained in the respiration chamber under reduced oxygen pressure in which the measurements were made with the hydrogen electrode by Parsons [15].

Subject	Place	Work km. per min.	Increase in pH	Place	Work km. per min.	Increase in pH
Redfield	Boston	750	·12	Cerro	193	·11
Barcroft	Cambridge	640	·08	Chamber	370	·08[1]

The mechanism of the increased breathlessness in exercise is pretty clear. The respiratory centre at high altitudes is more irritable on account of the want of oxygen, and therefore it reacts more violently to a given increment of hydrogen-ion concentration and in addition the increment of hydrogen-ion concentration resulting from a given quantity of exercise is greater, so that the breathlessness is the cumulative effect of the double cause.

But, as time goes on, a mitigating circumstance arises, namely, the blood becomes buffered to a greater degree. The evidence of this fact emerged for a series of determinations which were largely carried out by Bock and Binger. These determinations dealt with the CO_2 dissociation curve of the blood at low and high altitudes. The following considerations may be applied to the study of the curve:

(a) The buffering of the blood may be described as the change in acid content of the blood, in this case CO_2, for a given increment of acid, in reaction say 1×10^{-8}.

(b) The shape of the curve is represented over the physiological range by the equation

$$v\,CO_2 = a \times cH \times 10^8 + b,$$

where a and b are constants. Of these a represents the change in cH when the change in the volume of CO_2 is 1, and may therefore be taken as the numerical expression of the degree of buffering.

The following figures (31 and 32) show the change in CO_2 content for a change of 1×10^{-8} in the concentration of hydrogen-ions in:

(a) Meakins's blood at sea-level;

(b)   ,,   ,,   within a day or two of arrival at Cerro;

(c) Harrop's blood at sea-level;

(d)   ,,   ,,   after residence at Cerro.

In Meakins's case the buffer value corresponds to 6·7 c.c. of CO_2 for each increment of $1 \times 10^{-8} cH$ both before and just after reaching Cerro. In Harrop's case, which was confirmed by that of Binger, after a fortnight's residence at Cerro the quantity of CO_2 necessary to change the blood reaction by $1 \times 10^{-8} cH$ had risen from 5·5 to 7·5 c.c. This rise corresponds roughly to the rise in hæmoglobin content of the blood.

[1] The increment in cH is greater than the average value found by Arborelius and Liljestrand(16) but not greater than individual observations in their paper.

When one speaks of a given piece of exercise producing a given degree of dyspnœa, one is dealing really with a chain of events. This chain consists of at least three links, (1) the muscular mechanism in order to perform a given task may produce more or less acid, i.e., it may alter in efficiency; (2) the given increment of acid to the blood may produce a greater or less change in the hydrogen-ion concentra-

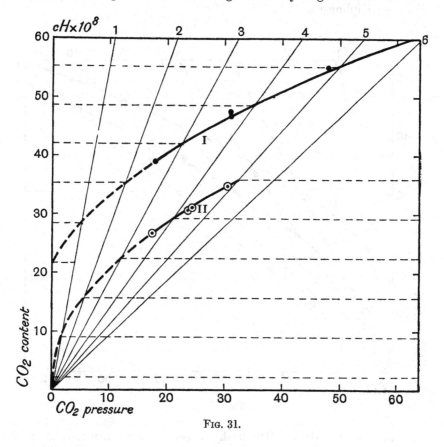

Fig. 31.

tion of the blood, i.e., the buffer-value of the blood may alter; and (3) a given change in the blood reaction may produce a greater or lesser change in the total ventilation, i.e., the irritability of the centre may alter. At Cerro all these factors underwent a change and they did not all change in the same direction. The first and third varied in such a way as to increase the tendency to dyspnœa, the second in such a way as to reduce it. Acclimatisation will be discussed in a later chapter, but the change in blood reaction—one factor only in acclimatisation—shows that the process is not a simple one, it comes more near to being a complete readjustment in which, as in a ship on her first voyage, the whole structure stretches a little here and shrinks a little there so that the strain is taken up equally by the whole fabric, after the fashion so graphically described by Rudyard Kipling(17).

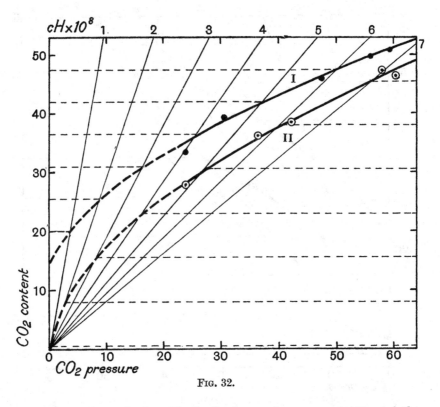

Fig. 32.

So far we have dealt with the hydrogen-ion concentration of the plasma, having only made a passing allusion to that of the corpuscles in order to indicate that the relation between the hydrogen-ion concentration of the corpuscles and that of the plasma might vary. The effect of any variation of the reaction on the inside of the corpuscle would be, other things being equal, to alter the affinity for oxygen of the hæmoglobin contained within the corpuscle wall. Thus, if the inside of the corpuscle becomes more alkaline, the hæmoglobin will be more retentive of its oxygen, if the inside of the corpuscle becomes more acid, the reverse will be the case.

This change in the affinity of hæmoglobin for oxygen may be produced experimentally in the following way, as was pointed out to me by Dr Cecil Murray (18). If a sample of blood N be shaken with air so that much of the CO_2 be driven out, it is to be expected from the work of Hamburger, that the chlorides will migrate to some extent from the interior of the corpuscle into the plasma, the bases remaining in the corpuscle. At this stage the blood is centrifuged and divided into two portions A and B, the one richer and the other poorer in corpuscles than the original. If, now, the portion A be taken and equilibrated with air containing the same pressure of CO_2 as that to which the blood was originally exposed, chlorides will return from the plasma into the corpuscles, but as the ratio of corpuscles to plasma is much greater than before, the amount of chloride which returns into each corpuscle is not nearly so great as that which came out and therefore the inside of the corpuscle will be relatively much more alkaline. If the sample B had been similarly treated, the reaction of the inside of the corpuscles would be more acid than originally. The repercussion of these changes in reaction would be that if (1) N, the original blood, (2) sample A, and (3) sample B, were equilibrated respectively with a given mixture of oxygen and carbonic acid, A would contain a greater percentage saturation and B a less percentage saturation of oxygen than the original blood, N.

The following example shows a comparison between A and N in which the hydrogen-ion concentration of the plasma is almost the same for both, as measured by the hydrogen electrode, but the affinity of the corpuscles for oxygen is widely different.

	Hæmoglobin value	pH of reduced blood at 27 mm. CO_2 pressure	Oxygen pressure	Percentage saturation with oxygen
Blood A	154	7·39	19	74
Blood N	108	7·36	19	34

These two bloods would of course have very different dissociation curves. If one draws the curves according to one of the accepted equations, through the two points which I have indicated in the above table, they come out as shown in Fig. 33.

Indeed Dr Uyeno (19) and I obtained quite similar curves by treating blood in the way which I have described.

The reason why the matter was of such interest to us is that our own oxygen dissociation curves underwent just such a change at Cerro de Pasco.

In Fig. 34, *a* to *c*, the actual quantities of oxygen which the blood contains (not the percentage saturations) are plotted as the ordinates and the oxygen pressures as the abscissæ, *a* refers to a sample of my blood, Curve I being the normal, Curve II being that of the blood if the corpuscles were simply concentrated in number so as to increase the hæmoglobin value 50 per cent., and Curve III, my blood,

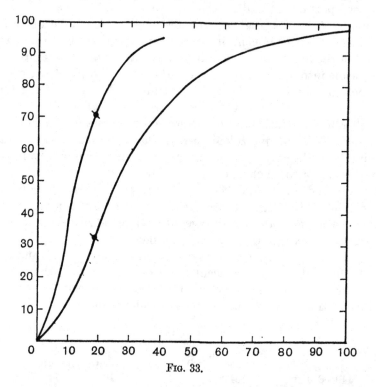

FIG. 33.

but treated in the way I have described for the sample *A* above, also concentrated so that it has a hæmoglobin value of 150. Fig. 34, *b*, Curve I is the normal dissociation curve of Binger, Curve II is what would be obtained if his blood simply contained enough corpuscles of the normal character to make his hæmoglobin value up to what was observed at Cerro, and Curve III is the actual curve which he had at Cerro. Curve III in Fig. 34, *c*, is that of a native at Cerro, we have

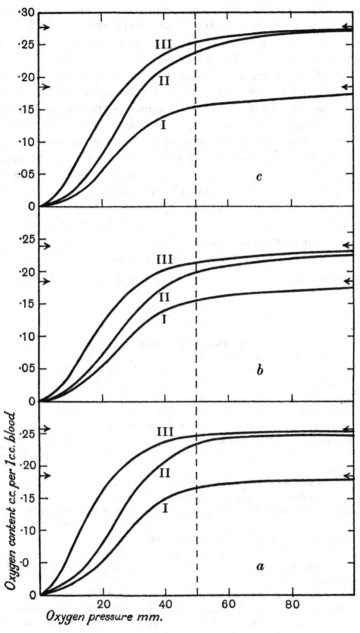

Fig. 34.

no sea-level curve of the same person with which to compare it. Therefore we have put on the same normal curve as in Fig. 34, *b*, and in Curve II we have magnified it up to the hæmoglobin value which was found in Villareal's blood.

In the figure there is a dotted line at 50 mm. oxygen pressure. This is about the pressure of the oxygen in the alveolar air at Cerro. The curves show that at such a pressure the arterial blood is appreciably more saturated than would otherwise be the case. The effect at Cerro however is only commencing to be well marked, if you go down to 25[1] mm. pressure, which is about what might be expected towards the top of Everest, the difference in oxygen content of the blood as between Curves II and III in either Fig. 34 *a*, *b* or *c* is very great, and without some such readjustment as enables the reaction in the corpuscle to become more alkaline, while that in the plasma remains approximately constant, man would probably have been confined to much lower levels than he has attained.

[1] Observations made at 23,000 feet by Somervell suggest that 25 mm. is too low. See Appendix.

BIBLIOGRAPHY

(1) BERT, PAUL. *La pression barométrique*. 1878.

(2) MOSSO, A. *Life of Man in the High Alps*, Chap. xxii. London, 1898.

(3) HENDERSON, YANDELL. Numerous papers in *American Journal of Physiol*. XXI.–XXV.

(4) BARCROFT. *Journ. Physiol.* XLII. 44. 1911.

(5) HALDANE AND PRIESTLEY. *Journ. Physiol.* XXXII. 225. 1905.

(6) LEWIS, COTTON, RYFFEL, WOLF AND BARCROFT. *Heart*, v. 52. 1913.

(7) FRASER, ROSS AND DREYER. *Quart. Journ. Med.* XV. 195. 1922.

(8) BARCROFT, CAMIS, MATHISON, ROBERTS AND RYFFEL. *Phil. Trans.* B. CCVI. 49. 1914.

(9) HENDERSON, YANDELL. *Science* (N.S.), XLIX. 431. 1910.

(10) HENDERSON AND HAGGARD. *Journ. of Biol. Chem.* XXI. 1919.

(11) KELLAS, KENNAWAY AND HALDANE. *Journ. Physiol.* LIII. 181. 1919.

(12) HASSELBALCH AND LINDHARD. *Biochem. Zeitsch.* LXVIII. 294. 1915.

(13) DALE AND EVANS. *Journ. Physiol.* LIV. 167. 1920.

(14) W. E. L. BROWN. Demonstrated to Physiological Society, March 1925.

(15) BARCROFT, PARSONS, T. R. AND PARSONS, W. *Physiol. Proc., Journ. Physiol.* LIII. CX. 1920.

(16) ARBORELIUS AND LILJESTRAND. *Skand. Arch.* XLIV. 215. 1923.

(17) RUDYARD KIPLING. "The Ship that Found Herself." *The Day's Work.* 1898.

(18) BARCROFT AND MURRAY. *Phil. Trans Roy. Soc.* B. CCXI. Appendices 2 and 3.

(19) BARCROFT AND UYENO. *Journ. Physiol.* LVII. 200. 1923.

CHAPTER VIII

THE PULSE

THERE has been much difference of opinion as to the effect of altitude upon the pulse. Some observers have said that the pulse rate is accelerated at high altitudes, others take the opposite view (1).

Since the publication of most of these observations a great deal has been found out about the pulse, and about the efficiency of the heart as judged by the pulse. The methods which we used in Peru reflect much of this work and are largely based on the conceptions with which Sir James Mackenzie and Sir Thomas Lewis have made us familiar. In view however of the conflicting statements which have been made, it seems worth while to preface this account of our own findings by some general discussion of the effect of oxygen want upon the pulse.

If the heart be taken out of an animal it may of course be kept beating for many hours by the maintenance of a suitable artificial circulation through the vessels of the coronary system. Among the essential ingredients of such a circulating fluid is oxygen. If the oxygen be cut off the beats become less frequent and finally cease. At no stage is there an acceleration of the heart beat due to lack of oxygen supply. The direct result of want of oxygen on the heart itself is slowing.

The remarkable tracing shown in Fig. 35 indicates the effect of asphyxia in the heart of an animal which is just dying from failure of the respiratory centre. Here it will be seen that not only do the beats become "fewer and farther between" but that they alter in character, the principal alteration being a lengthening of that particular portion known to cardiologists as the $P - R$ interval, which represents the length of time taken by the impulse to pass from the sino-auricular node to the auriculo-ventricular node.

In connection with a study of experimental aortic regurgitation it was shown by Sands[1] (Bazett's pupil) that when asphyxia was

---

[1] Preliminary report at Edinburgh, Eleventh International Congress. Data given in a personal communication.

produced late in chloroform anæsthesia there was a slowing of the conduction rate. Thus in Dog No. 3:

	P.-R.	Q.-R.-S.
Normal	·140 sec.	·036 sec.
Immediately after producing an aortic lesion	·123	·026
Twelve weeks later	·148	·055
Early chloroform anæsthesia	·135	·077
Late chloroform anæsthesia	·147	·059
	·176	·078
	·193	·071
	·251	·077
After respiration had ceased	·284	·087
	·340	·107
	·588	·151
	—	·229

This lengthening of conduction time may be taken as the hall-mark of an asphyxiated heart, in the absence of an anatomical lesion.

The effect of want of oxygen on the pulse in the living animal has been studied by many observers, the most recent of whom perhaps are Charles W. Greene and N. C. Gilbert [2]. The result of such observations has been to show that in the living animal the effect of anoxæmia on the pulse is quite different from anything which could have been predicted by a study of the excised heart—whether excised actually or functionally.

We may here throw out a word of caution to the reader. It will be necessary for him to follow rather closely the time relation of the events which are recounted. There is no assumption that the effect of sudden deprivation of oxygen will be the same as that of gradual deprivation, or that an anoxæmia which produces a fatal effect in a matter of hours can be compared to one which leaves the subject acclimatised after some days.

Greene and Gilbert performed experiments in which dogs were subjected to a gradual deprivation of oxygen which was obtained by allowing dogs to re-breathe their own expired air, the CO_2 being removed from the same. The anoxæmia crept on at a rate which allowed about four hours' rebreathing before a fatal result supervened. During the earlier part of the four hours the respirations became more rapid until a critical point was reached, after which the respiratory centre commenced to fail. This point Greene and Gilbert call the respiratory crisis and their observations show that in the type of anoxæmia which they established, the pulse follows the respirations fairly closely. Unlike anything which takes place in the excised heart, the pulse quickens as the result of anoxæmia. The quickening becomes more marked up to, but only up to, the moment of the respiratory crisis. After that the pulse, as in the excised heart, commences to fail.

Greene and Gilbert's experiments were undertaken for the American Air Force. A much less complete series undertaken for the British Gas Warfare Organisation (3) which differed from those of Greene and Gilbert in that we precipitated the crisis with great suddenness and completeness—(sometimes with a result immediately fatal)—by imposing considerable muscular contractions upon the animal.

The essential difference—from the present point of view—between

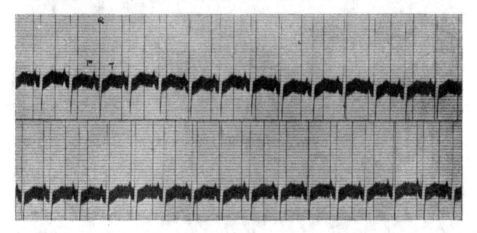

FIG. 35, *a*. Normal rabbit, rest.

an animal which has been gassed and one that has not, is that in the former case there is a slight deficiency of oxygen in the resting animal and a considerable deficiency of oxygen as soon as exercise is taken. Into the theory of this we have already gone (see Fig. 22). I am now speaking of an animal severely but not fatally gassed with a pulmonary irritant such as phosgene. In such an animal the effect of exercise is just the opposite from what it is in a normal animal. Exercise quickens the normal pulse, but in the anoxæmic animal exercise may slow the previously rapid pulse and even stop it.

The slowing which is associated with muscular contraction in the anoxæmic has nothing in common with that which has already been described as due to asphyxia of the heart. The crisis precipitated by exercise is the result of something which takes place in the brain.

It appears to be an intense stimulation of the vagus nerve. The story is told in the tracings. Fig. 35, *a* and *b*, are two electrocardiograms from a normal rabbit, *a* at rest, and *b* when it was made to kick about by irritation with electric shocks. The pulse in *a* is slower (about 230) than that in *b* (about 270). The rabbit was gassed

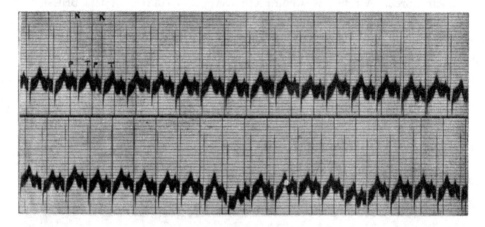

FIG. 35, *b*. Normal rabbit; muscular exercise.

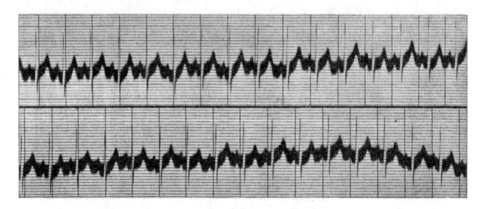

FIG. 35, *c*. Same rabbit two days after being gassed, rest.

six days subsequently and on the seventh day records again were taken. Fig. 35, record *c*, is from the resting rabbit. It is worth noting the resemblance between records *c* and *b*, i.e., between the resting gassed, and the exercised normal animal. The resemblance may be observed in two particulars: (1) the rate (about 270 in *b* and 300 in *c*), and (2) the exaggeration of the T-wave in each as compared with *a*.

After taking record *c* we were about to take one in which the animal was again stimulated and made to kick about, but it forestalled us. On being taken up it struggled and respiration ceased. Fig. 35, record *d*, shows what was happening—or rather not happening in the heart—the heart "stopped dead," the beats ceasing completely

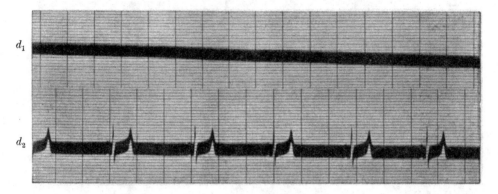

FIG. 35, *d*. Rabbit similar to *a–c*. Muscular exercise causes death;
d_1 = moment of death.

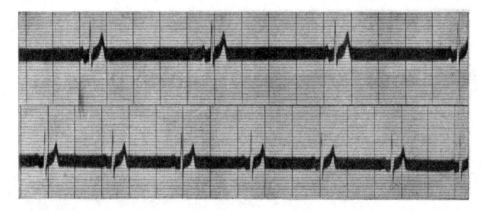

FIG. 35, *e*.

for the time. But it was only for the time; once the animal was really dead, that is to say, once the heart was free from the control of the nervous system, it again commenced to beat, and the subsequent tracings, Fig. 35, d_2, *e* and *f*, were taken at intervals up to seven minutes after death.

It has already been stated that a lengthening of the conduction time is the index of asphyxiation of the heart itself. Let us examine the records in the light of this statement.

As compared with record a, there is no sign of asphyxiation in b or c. In d_1 there are no beats to study and in d_2 the $P - R$ interval

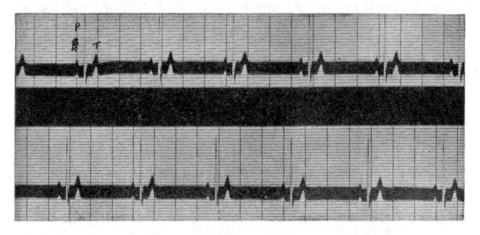

FIG. 35, f. Four minutes after death.

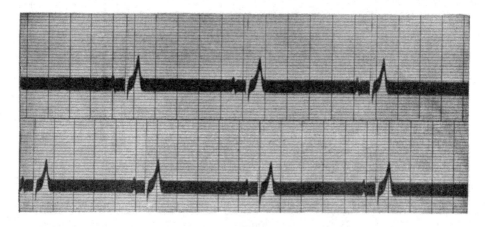

FIG. 35, g. Seven minutes after death.

is no longer than in a or c. Therefore up to and after the death of the animal there was no sign of actual want of oxygen by the heart itself, but the sign soon appears, for in the subsequent tracings the $P - R$ interval gradually lengthens out till in record g it extends over more than one-tenth of a second. Granting then that in record d_1

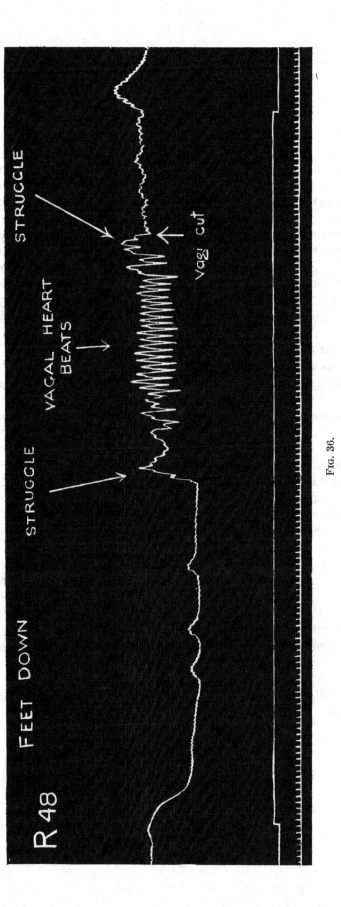

Fig. 36.

(Fig. 35), the cause of stoppage is not oxygen want on the part of the heart itself, the alternative cause would naturally be vagus stimulation, of which there is independent evidence as follows.

When struggling takes place under anoxæmic conditions the associated slowing of the heart does not always amount to complete stoppage. In such cases it is possible by cutting the vagi to restore the previous rapid pulse. A record of the phenomenon may be observed in the tracing given on p. 109. It is a tracing of the arterial pressure in a rabbit which was suffering from phosgene poisoning and it consists of three portions: (1) before the commencement of struggling, (2) immediately after struggling, (3) during a second period of struggling, the opportunity being seized to cut the vagi. It will be seen that the slow vagal cardiac rhythm associated with the muscular effort is exchanged for the original rapid pulse.

Let us sum up the position so far as we have discussed it before proceeding to consider what actually happens at high altitudes.

The effect of oxygen want on the heart itself is to slowing and ultimate stoppage. The effect has, as far as I know, never been observed at high altitudes, for before the anoxæmia is so profound as to produce it the central nervous system will be "down and out." Certainly in athletic men one may disregard it. We are left then to consider the effect of oxygen want on the cardiac centre, or centres, in the medulla. This would appear to be in the resting animal entirely in the direction of quickening the heart until the central nervous system itself commences to lose its grip. The extent to which the quickening is due to loss of vagus control or to increase of sympathetic control I am not in a position to discuss. With all moderate amounts of anoxæmia then one may look for a quickening of the heart. There is no reason why this should not apply to exercise as well as to rest, but muscular exercise may provoke a vagal reaction under circumstances as yet but ill-defined, a vagal reaction which would appear to be best marked in profound anoxæmia and which in cases where the respiratory centre is "on its last legs" it may prove fatal.

Now to pass to the mountains.

The following are some pulse records taken in the train going up the Central Railway of Peru (4).

Place			Altitude	Pulse
Tamborague	...	...	9,826	64
San Matteo	...	...	10,534	74
Rio Blanco	...	...	11,430	78

It is entirely in keeping with the mental altitude of the high mountains that above Casapalca (13,606 feet), at which height the patient "began to feel really bad with a good vigorous headache and a slight feeling of nausea," and when therefore the pulse would have been really interesting, no records were taken. We may supply them from the researches of Schneider and Truesdell, who show that the heart rate increases by 20 beats when the pressure drops to that corresponding to 18,000 feet (5).

There is no doubt then that the effect of altitude above 10,000 feet on resting persons who are not acclimatised is to quicken the pulse. The acclimatised person presents a somewhat different problem. Let us start with his basal pulse after a sufficient residence at Cerro to produce acclimatisation. There is no evidence that altitude up to 14,000 feet has any certain effect upon it.

Pulses under Basal Conditions

Name	Place	Pulse	Pulse at Cerro
Meakins	ss. *Victoria*	63	60–63
	ss. *Victoria*	63	—
Barcroft	ss. *Victoria*	60	58
	ss. *Victoria*	64	—
Bock	Lima	60	61
Binger	Lima	60	60
Redfield	Lima	57	65
	—	—	59
Harrop	Lima	58	62

In the case of the first two subjects, great care was taken that the conditions should be quite uniform. The pulse was always counted by another person, and at certain periods in a basal metabolism experiment. Our idea was that not only should the body be as free as possible from effort, but the mind as free as possible from thought. The experiments took place about 7 a.m. Everything was prepared by the observer, the subject was then waked, if, as was usual, he was still asleep, and the experiment commenced with no exercise of mind or body on the part of the subject. The figures given are the mean usually of three or four counts.

There is but one conclusion to be drawn, namely that the facts do not justify any such statement as that the pulse at Cerro de Pasco is more rapid than at the sea-level. On one or two cases it was so, never to any marked extent—on other cases the reverse was the case. Note that we are speaking now about the basal as distinct from the ordinary resting pulse.

Whether the same would be true at altitudes of a higher order than 14,000 to 15,000 feet we do not know[1], but it is to be supposed that had we made similar researches at higher altitudes each one of us would eventually have reached some altitude at which the oxygen want would have been sufficient to quicken the pulse, even under conditions of the utmost rest of which the body was capable. Much confusion has arisen from a lack of specific statement of the actual altitude at which changes commence to take place and a lack of recognition of the fact that the critical altitude for one person will be different from that for another. Granting then that we take the basal pulse as our starting point, what is the effect of exertion?

The method by which we tested the influence of exercise on the pulse was different from that used heretofore by the Alpine observers. It was similar to that recently introduced for the testing of soldiers and now used largely in England by insurance companies.

The precise detail of the test was furnished to us by Dr G. H. Hunt of Guy's Hospital. As carried out by Hunt, the subject mounts a stool one-third of a metre in height a given number of times, in each three instances the number increasing as the exercise becomes more exacting. The exercise extends over three minutes in each case. The pulse is taken at rest before each exercise and for the two minutes immediately succeeding each exercise. The post-exercise pulse rate is divided by the resting pulse rate and an index is obtained. For example

	Exercise		Resting pulse two minutes	Post exercise pulse	Index
	No. of steps in three mins.	Kilogram metres			
I	36	1800	146	84 + 78	1·11
II	54	2700	140	89 + 78	1·19
III	72	3600	138	108 + 83	1·38
IV	90	4500	140	130 + 105	1·67

A graph is then constructed in which the index is the ordinate and the severity of the exercise, either expressed in steps or kilogram metres, is the abscissa. In this way the amount of work which can be done before a certain index is reached can be ascertained.

At Cerro we varied the method to the extent that instead of using the resting pulse as obtained in the sitting posture we used the basal as the denominator of the index. In the construction of the following

[1] See Appendix I.

graph therefore the 62 used is the basal pulse at the sea level and the 58 that at Cerro de Pasco.

The response of the pulse at sea-level to the exercises stated, is shown by the black dots which represent observations made on the ss. *Victoria*. At Chosica (2700 feet) the response clearly does not differ (circle) from that at the sea-level. At Cerro de Pasco, however, the response to exercise is quite different, a much smaller degree of exercise (about two-thirds of the amount) being necessary to produce a given response.

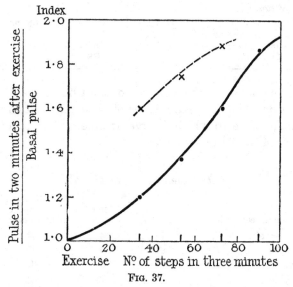

Fig. 37.

Quite similar results were obtained with regard to Meakins's pulse.

Had the above figure been drawn from indices obtained by taking the resting pulse as the divisor instead of the basal pulse little difference would have been seen between the curves at Cerro and at sea-level, the "resting" pulses being accelerated in about the same proportions as the exercise pulses.

One set of observations which appeared to be anomalous is of interest as it brought out a special feature of the pulse. Whether the appearance of this feature was accidental or whether it would always appear if the subject went to the same altitude from sea-level could only be determined by a course of experiments. At Matucana (7700 feet) Barcroft in the second minute after exercise experienced

B

a marked bradycardia. The following were the figures obtained from successive exercises:

Exercise Steps	I 36	II 54	III 72
Matucana			
Pulse at rest	67, 66	66, 67	65, 66
Pulse after exercise			
1st minute	75	80	90
2nd minute	62	67	74
ss. *Victoria*			
Pulse at rest	64, 64	64, 65	68, 68
Pulse after exercise			
1st minute	79	98	—
2nd minute	69	79	—

I have to thank two of the members of the 1924 Everest expedition for information about the pulse rates of their party at much higher altitudes than those to which I have attained. The following data are given by Major Hingston:

Pulse rate of one individual

Altitude in feet	Sitting	Standing	After exercise	Time in seconds of return of pulse to normal
Sea-level	72	72	84	20
7,000	72	84	96	15
14,300	72	84	105	40
16,500	72	96	120	20
21,000	108	120	144	20

The points in the above table which seem to me to form an interesting criticism on our own observations are: (1) from the first column it appears that there was no rise in the pulse when sitting until above a height of 16,500 feet, higher than that a rise took place; (2) the greater the amount of exercise, the lower was the level at which altitude affected the pulse; (3) in the last column, at 7000 feet, there was an abnormally rapid return to the normal, no doubt the vagal phenomenon which we observed at the same height.

Dr Somervell in a memorandum sent to me says: "In the neighbourhood of 27,000 to 28,000 feet...the heart during actual motion upwards was found to be beating at 160 to 180 per minute, sometimes even more; regular in rhythm and of good volume."

BIBLIOGRAPHY

(1) The bibliography of the older work will be found in Mosso's *Life in the High Alps*; Zuntz, Loewy, Müller and Caspari's *Höhenklima und Bergwanderungen*, Berlin, 1906; Schneider's article in Vol. I of *Physiological Reviews*.

(2) GREENE AND GILBERT. *Amer. Journ. Physiol.* LX. 155. 1922.

(3) *Chemical Warfare Medical Committee Report*, No. XIV.

(4) BARCROFT, BINGER, BOCK, DOGGART, FORBES, HARROP, MEAKINS AND REDFIELD. *Phil. Trans.* B. CCXI. 351. 1923.

(5) SCHNEIDER. *Physiol. Reviews*, I. 652. 1921.

CHAPTER IX

THE CIRCULATION RATE

In forms of expression of a rhetorical character such as advertisements or sermons one often sees some course of treatment or effort of chivalry recommended on grounds such as the following: it heightens the colour in the cheeks, it makes the pulse beat faster and causes the blood to circulate more rapidly through the vessels. Let us lay aside the sermons for the time being and confine ourselves to the advertisements. A friend of mine once remarked that the art of successful advertisement consisted in making some statement about the commodity advertised which was in fact perfectly true but which was quite irrelevant. Ever since that piece of wisdom was poured in my ears I have been unable to avoid the scrutiny of advertisements from this particular point of view. I say to myself, granting that the statement in this or that advertisement is true, does it really matter? Will the person be any better for having the colour in his cheeks heightened, for having a more rapid pulse, and having a greater quantity of blood coursing through his vessels? Or to put the matter in more technical language, is one better for having an increased minute volume, by which is meant an increased volume of blood passing each minute from the right to the left side of the heart through the lungs and from the left to the right through the general circulation?

The rhetorician of course uses these three expressions—the heightening of the colour, the quickening of the pulse and the increase of minute volume—as though they were merely three different ways of expressing the same thing. Such an hypothesis could not be accepted without enquiry—and later we will investigate the validity of the assumption that an increase of the pulse rate implies an increase of output of the heart per minute. At the moment, however, I want to take up the question whether it may be regarded as an advantage to the individual to have a large minute volume, and in particular whether it is of advantage at an altitude of 14,000 feet.

Let us take the more general question first. We can measure the quantity of blood which traverses the circulation in a minute, roughly perhaps, but yet with sufficient exactitude to enable us to appraise the relevance of his statements. The principles on which such measurements can be carried out are best illustrated by a reference to experiments upon animals, since the methods applied to animals are simpler and the description of the principles less complicated by details.

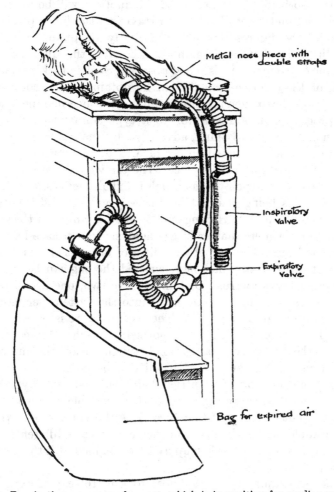

Metal nose piece with double straps

Inspiratory valve

Expiratory valve

Bag for expired air

FIG. 38. Respiration apparatus for goat, which is in position for cardiac puncture.

The argument is as follows: the animal absorbs a certain quantity of oxygen each minute into its system. This oxygen passes from the air in its lungs through the lung epithelium and is absorbed by the blood. Clearly if the amount of oxygen each cubic centimetre of blood absorbs is measured and the resulting figure is multiplied by the number of cubic centimetres of blood which pass through the lung in a minute, the product indicates the total quantity of oxygen taken up. Or, to put this matter in another way, if this total quantity of oxygen taken up (which we will call Q) is divided by the quantity which is absorbed by 1 c.c. of blood the quotient will be the number of cubic centimetres of blood which traversed the lungs per minute.

There are two figures to be obtained, firstly, the quantity of oxygen which the animal uses per minute, secondly, the quantity which each cubic centimetre of his blood absorbs. Such is Fick's[1] method.

Each of these measurements can be obtained with comparative ease. So far as the oxygen used by the animal is concerned the following is the procedure[2]. A respirator, of a type similar to that used in the French army and, I think, advocated by the American army at the end of the war, is fitted on the face. Fig. 38 shows a goat lying down with the respirator in place. The air which it inhales enters the respirator at one point, that which it exhales leaves it at another (both apertures being guarded by one way valves) and the expired air is collected in a bag. Having once secured a sample of the expired air it becomes a mere matter of gas analysis to estimate how much oxygen has been taken out of each litre of atmospheric air and the number of litres of air which have entered the bag can be measured by means of a gas metre. Combining these two, one arrives at the amount of oxygen the goat absorbed into the system per minute—this is the first figure, namely Q. The second figure is obtained very simply. The amount of oxygen absorbed by each cubic centimetre of blood is the difference in saturation between the arterial and venous bloods respectively, samples of blood can be obtained by cardiac puncture, the right or left ventricle being entered by a hypodermic needle attached to a syringe. It is then possible to measure the oxygen content of each. If therefore A be the volume of oxygen in the arterial blood and V be that in the venous—the difference $A - V$ is the quantity of oxygen taken up by 1 c.c. of blood, it is the measurement R.

To take an example: a certain goat took in 160 c.c. of oxygen per minute (that is $Q = 160$),

1 c.c. arterial blood contained	·117 c.c. of oxygen.
1 c.c. venous ,, ,,	·060 ,,
Oxygen absorbed by c.c. of blood	·057 c.c. = R.

$$\frac{Q}{R} = \frac{160}{·057} = 2632 \text{ c.c. or 2·6 litres.}$$

The method of measurement is more difficult in man, the reason being that the procedure necessary to obtain an average sample of venous blood though extremely simple might, if it miscarried, be dangerous. Therefore a rather complicated method of making the measurement of oxygen in the venous blood indirectly has been introduced.

The method used, and one which I think was then the best, was worked out by Dr Redfield, Dr Bock and Prof. Meakins[3], based on methods previously in existence.

The principle is as follows: the air in the lungs comes into equilibrium with the blood which comes from the heart and the composition of that air can be investigated, then from known data one can calculate the composition of the blood with which the air was in equilibrium.

The difficulty which the authors surmounted, however, lies in the fact that the air in the lungs does not come into complete equilibrium with the venous blood which comes from the heart. This difficulty was met in the following manner: if from a bag one inhales a sample of air and breathes out half of it, and then after ten or fifteen seconds the remaining half is forced out, the latter half will be more nearly in equilibrium with the venous blood than the former half. By plotting the quantities of oxygen and carbonic acid in the two samples on a graph (see page 34), the one as the ordinate and the other as the abscissa, two points are obtained and if the line which joins them be extended it will indicate the location of a point where there would be equilibrium between the alveolar air and the venous blood. The operation is repeated, the bag being filled with an atmosphere of quite different composition, another line is then obtained which will also point to the final position of equilibrium and by again altering the composition of the inspired air a third line is obtained.

Dr Redfield, Dr Bock and Prof. Meakins found that frequently the successive lines all crossed at a certain point. When that was the case there was but one conclusion, namely, that this point registered the composition of an atmosphere which would have been in equilibrium with the venous blood. Having discovered such a point, the amount of oxygen there would be in 1 c.c. of blood, which was in equilibrium with such air, can be determined, if one has knowledge of the hæmoglobin value of the subject and uses capillary dissociation curve[4]. The above method is given in some detail because it is the method which we used, out of it grew that of E. K. Marshall and myself (5), which is much simpler and which I should now use[1].

The arterial blood can be obtained by puncture of the radial artery, and at high altitudes this must be done. At sea-level it may be assumed to be 95 per cent. saturated. Hence we have the data for calculating R. Q is obtained precisely as in the goat.

Having explained so much about the method let me now revert to the enquiry regarding the desirability of having a rapid blood flow. Such information as we have on the subject comes from the writings of Prof. Krogh of Copenhagen (7). Prof. Krogh's view is that in persons of fine bodily development and of superior physical capability such as athletes, the blood flow relative to their metabolism is slow. Thus in an athletic man the blood flow at rest was 3·4 litres per minute, while in his wife it was half as much again. The construction which Krogh put on this rather surprising phenomenon was directly deducible from the principles which we have already enumerated. For a given value of Q, the smaller the minute volume the greater must be the value of R in the equation

$$\text{Min. Vol.} = \frac{Q}{R}.$$

That is to say the smaller the blood flow the more oxygen is taken from the blood at each circuit of the body and therefore the more efficient the system, inasmuch as a quieter circulation suffices to supply a given quantity of oxygen to the body. There is no doubt that in the case of our own party the results bear out Prof. Krogh's.

---

[1] The history of these methods has undergone rather an interesting evolution. Based on the work of Christiansen, Douglas and Haldane a method was put forward by Haldane and Douglas (6) in which a sample of a gas mixture of oxygen CO_2 and nitrogen was inspired, an alveolar sample rapidly given out and another after a short interval. If these two were identical in their content both of oxygen and CO_2 the sample was taken as being in equilibrium with the mixed venous blood. In practice this method suffered from the same objection as that of triple extrapolation, namely, that in between the intervals of breathing various gas mixtures the minute volume might change. Haldane and Douglas therefore applied an empirical correction which was that if the oxygen readings from their two samples differed by only a little, that difference added to the oxygen in the second sample gave the true reading, i.e., if the oxygens were 32 and 34 mm. respectively the true reading would be 36 mm. If Barcroft and Marshall's figures (e.g., Figs. 1 and 3) be examined it will be seen that the same is true of the oxygen readings in these figures also, both sets of observers starting from different premises have arrived at an identical method. Therefore the true reading may be obtained from the very simple technique of Barcroft and Marshall by adding to the second oxygen reading the difference between the second and first.

Unfortunately I would have to yield the palm for physical efficiency, without a struggle, either to Dr Redfield or to Prof. Meakins. Our circulation rates as determined by the method of triple extrapolation are as follows:

Barcroft	Meakins	Redfield
6·8 ⎫	4·9 ⎫	
5·4 ⎬ 6·1	4·4 ⎪	4·2
6·0 ⎭	5·5 ⎬ 5·1	
	5·4 ⎭	

Personally I see the matter from rather a different angle, namely, that of the amount of margin which the heart and circulatory system have to draw upon in case of emergency, say heavy exercise. Let us assume that Prof. Meakins's heart and my own are each capable of an output of 19 litres per minute—my heart at rest is putting out about one-third of that amount and his about one-fourth, therefore he can speed up his circulation to four times its present volume per minute, I can only speed up mine to three times.

Two criticisms may legitimately be made of the above argument:

(1) Is it a justifiable assumption that Prof. Meakins's heart is capable of as great an output per minute as my own? It is difficult to say of what a person's heart may be capable when divorced from the body in which it is. But considering Meakins's age and physique there can be no doubt that he is capable of a much more intense degree of physical exertion, i.e., a much greater oxygen absorption per minute. I have spoken of 19 litres of blood per minute, the whole amount of oxygen in that would be a little over three litres. I think that is an underestimate of what Meakins is capable of. I should be sorry nowadays to put the matter to the test on myself.

(2) The case of a person having a low output at rest which was incapable of being increased to any extent has been put to me in the following words: "Also the opposite case might be stated that a group of circumstances is possible under which a low output at rest is assumed which does not increase much with exercise—say only from 3 litres per minute at rest to 4·5 during exercise. Because the utilisation is already great and the increase of rate of flow is not great the oxygen debt will be relatively greater. Granted that Prof. Meakins may have a greater efficiency than you; yet you have a greater efficiency than such a case." Of course I agree, but a man of Meakins or even my development whose heart is only capable of a 4·5 litre per minute volume, could only absorb 750 c.c. of oxygen

per minute and would be pathological. Later I will quote the case of a patient who in attacks of paroxysmal tachycardia had a pulse of about 200 associated with a minute volume of two or three litres. He was incapable of any considerable exertion presumably because his heart was so inefficient.

The argument I developed above had reference to the really fit. Ruskin has said that the poor of this world are the entirely good and the entirely bad—or words to that effect. Possibly the persons with very low minute volumes are the really fit and the really unfit. At all events I must break with the rhetorician if he tries to persuade me that a large minute volume at rest is a desirable attribute—it seems rather to be an unnecessary evil. Even if a large minute volume may be of no advantage under ordinary circumstances, it may be that a speeding up of the circulation is extremely beneficial under conditions where the pressure of oxygen in the blood is abnormally low. Let us examine whether or not such an acceleration takes place at high altitudes.

We have seen that the blood, when it leaves the lung, lacks its full quotum of oxygen, firstly the pressure is deficient and secondly it may be that it is like an electric current which has fallen short of the proper voltage. One possible means of correcting this deficiency would be to force a greater quantity of blood through the tissues. The argument being that if the current has not enough volts the necessary power can be obtained by increasing the amperage. Of course it is a sort of scheme for substituting quantity for quality which is always unsatisfactory. On general grounds, however, it was to be expected, but general grounds apart, there were experimental data which pointed in the same direction. Some years ago Dr Dixon and I performed some experiments, as also did Starling and Markwalder [8], in which the circulation through the blood vessels of the heart was measured, while at the same time the oxygen in the blood which reached the heart was reduced.

On sufficient reduction of the oxygen in the arterial blood, the amount of blood which passed through the vessels of the heart muscle (coronary vessels) was increased, so that indeed the actual quantity of oxygen which reached the heart did not alter greatly regardless of wide variations in the quantity of oxygen in the arterial blood.

Fig. 39 is the hospital chart of a goat for some days after it had been gassed with phosgene [9]. Unlike most hospital charts, the items

	O₂ in arterial blood	Blood traversing heart per minute	Oxygen reaching heart
I	16 c.c. per cent.	11 c.c.	1·76
	14	11	1·54
	8	23	1·74
II	12	1·8	·21
	5·4	5·7	·31
III	15	8	1·20
	2·1	48	1·0

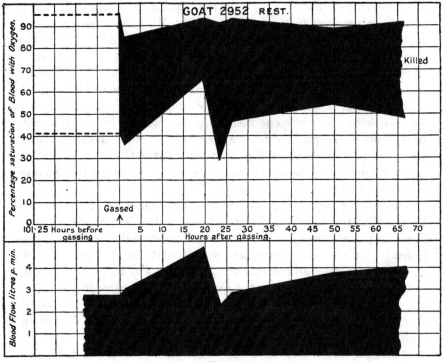

FIG. 39.

plotted are not the temperature, the respirations and pulse, but they are the oxygen in the arterial blood, the oxygen in the venous blood and the minute volume. The oxygen in the arterial blood is the top of the upper black area, the oxygen in the venous blood is the bottom of the same. The vertical height of the area represents the oxygen utilisation, i.e., the difference between the two. This is the figure (alluded to as R on page 118). The total oxygen absorbed per minute is not shown. From this data the minute volume is calculated which is represented by the lower black area. The result is typical of a great many though not of all cases of acute phosgene poisoning. We must pass over the problem of absorbing interest, namely, the reason why some goats like some persons react much more completely to poisons showing a more typical picture. The point with which we are concerned here is as follows. Are the successive changes in the minute volume caused by insufficient oxygen in the arterial blood? Was the initial rise in the minute volume a compensation in order to supply the tissues with a greater quantity of oxygen and thus to maintain the average pressure of oxygen in the capillary in spite of the drop of oxygen pressure in the arterial blood? Was the subsequent fall in the minute volume due to failure of the heart and if so was the heart failure due to deficient oxygen in the blood? These matters were of urgent interest during the war for if the cause were deficiency of oxygen the treatment indicated was the breathing of oxygen at high pressure. Their interest did not cease when the war ended because, after all, phosgene poisoning was merely an inflammation of the lung uncomplicated by the toxine of a bacillus and it therefore became a question whether the mechanical bar to the entry of oxygen into the blood, wrought by the œdema, was responsible for the changes observed in the minute volume.

Compare for instance goat 2952 at the termination of the experiment with 2150 which died after 34 hours. The two charts have in common the narrowing of the black area which indicates the utilisation up to about the eighteenth or nineteenth hour, then came in each case the large drop in the oxygen content of the venous blood, but there is this great difference at that critical period: in goat 2952 the oxygen content of the arterial blood was maintained, in 2150 it was not. Could goat 2150 have been saved if oxygen had been administered artificially at the eighteenth hour?

It seemed very desirable to test directly whether or not deficiency of oxygen in the arterial blood increased the minute volume, when the oxygen in the blood was reduced by cutting down the percentage of oxygen in the inspired air. This was undertaken by Dr Doi[10] and carried out with the greatest care, his result is the more convincing to me because it was obtained in the face of the greatest possible scepticism on my part.

The principal facts are shown in Fig. 43. Here the pulse rate (a circle) the minute volume (a dot) and the systolic output (a cross) are shown as percentages of the normal for the animal in question when breathing atmospheric air (21 per cent. oxygen).

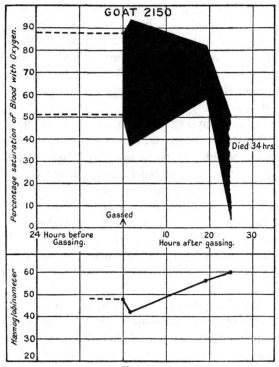

FIG. 40.

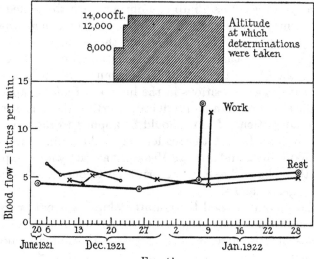

FIG. 41.

In no case did Doi obtain an increased minute volume when the cat breathed an atmosphere which was deficient in oxygen, the general trend of the results was in the opposite direction, though not very markedly so. Down to 13 per cent. oxygen in the inspired air (corresponding to an altitude of about 13,000 feet) the minute volume was over 90 per cent. of its original value. The issue was now raised in an acute form.

The results obtained by Doi on urethane cats could not be regarded as valid for unanæsthetised goats, or else the increase of the circulation rate in goats which was occasioned by phosgene poisoning was not due to anoxæmia and could not be regarded as a direct compensatory mechanism. This is the sort of problem that one does not lightly drop; there was no other alternative than test the effect of oxygen want on man himself, so away to the Andes!

The results which we brought home from Cerro were all too scanty and indeed they differed slightly according as to the method of observation employed. Two methods were used: (1) the method which I have described as that of triple extrapolation, the other a method which was devised independently by Meakins and Davies [11].

I must leave the reader to make up his own mind as to which method most nearly represents the facts and therefore I will give the results obtained by both methods, without prejudice. My own bias is naturally towards the triple extrapolation method because it is a fundamental article in my creed that in 15 seconds or so you cannot get any mixture of gas that you may inhale into equilibrium with the mixed venous blood. You may get a mixture of air and carbonic acid which you can breathe in and out without changing the quantity of CO_2 in the mixture. This is the basis of Meakins's method, but I think it only means that the CO_2 in the gas inhaled is churned up with a mixture of airs of varying compositions in the lung and that the appearance of an artificial equilibrium is produced. Further there is a question as to what corrections, if any, should be applied to the CO_2 reading when it is obtained. But the reader may hold a different view, as indeed Meakins does, and after all Meakins has vastly more experience of the method than I have. To return then to our results. They are shown in Figs. 42 and 43.

According to one method the minute volume was not appreciably altered as between the sea-level and Cerro de Pasco, according to the other it was slightly increased. The figures are as follows, taking the mean results:

Method of triple extrapolation

			Redfield	Meakins
Sea-level	...	...	5·1	5·2
Cerro ...	...	...	4·1	4·7

Meakins's method

Sea-level	...	...	5·3	7·8
Cerro ...	...	...	6·4	9·6

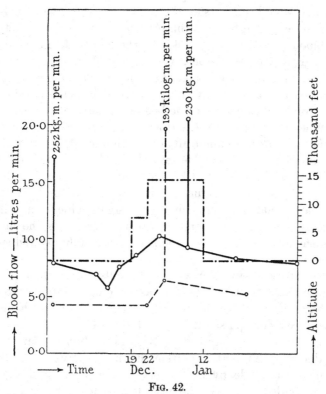

FIG. 42.

According to our method the blood fell about 20 per cent. or less, according to the other it rose about the same amount. It seems probable that there was very little change and certain that there was no *great* compensatory change. How trifling the change was, if any, may be gathered from the effect registered as the result of doing quite light work on the bicycle ergometer. Thus by Meakins's method 252 km. per minute caused in Edinburgh an increase of 9 to 10 litres per minute, whilst at Cerro 230 km. per minute caused an increase of 12 litres.

Of course, it will be clear to the reader that even if there is no increase in the volume of blood which passes round the "body-as-a-whole" it by no means follows that particular organs may not have an augmented supply. There may be a re-distribution and the brain might receive an augmented supply at the expense, for instance, of the skin. Indeed the blood supply of the brain might probably be greatly augmented without any change in the minute volume of the body which would fall outside the region of experimental error.

At Cerro we attempted some observations, by Stewart's method (12), on the blood flow through the skin of the hands. These were carried out with great care by Forbes, who estimated the rate at which the hand of a person in bed lost heat, but they yielded little information, the effect of altitude, if any, being marked by such considerations as the number of blankets on the bed of the subject.

Dr Schneider (13) in his excellent article on high altitude physiology in *Physiological Reviews* made an observation on Doi's research which has remained in my mind. He said that if Doi's work were correct the quickening of the heart at high altitudes would not be a compensatory mechanism but a signal of distress. For if the blood put out by the heart remains unaugmented that organ achieves nothing that is of use to the organism, and in Doi's experiments the heart did *quicken*, the systolic output becoming correspondingly reduced (see Fig. 37).

Yet the 20 per cent. increase in the pulse rate which prompted the phrase "signal of distress" is as nothing compared to effects which have been observed on men. Thus Haldane, Kellas and Kennaway (14) record pulse rates up to 120 under reduced atmospheric pressure in the steel chamber at Brompton, but by far the most remarkable and illuminating statement which I have come across on this subject was made by Dr Somervell at a meeting of the Royal Society of Medicine at which he described some of the experiences of the 1922[1] Everest Expedition. Quoting it from memory it was substantially as follows: "On the day of my highest climb" (he reached about 27,000 feet without oxygen) "my pulse went at about 200 most of the time." This indeed was a signal of distress! We know only a little about what happens to the minute volume when the heart goes at this sort of speed. The little we do know will be found in a paper (15) on a case of paroxysmal tachycardia. The patient—a

[1] Note, however, that Somervell says of the 1924 Expedition that the pulse "was of good volume."

student—happened to be a good physiologist and an excellent observer, so that he was able to give reasonably reliable data for the study of his own case. The result of observation of the minute volume during two attacks showed not merely that the tremendous acceleration of the pulse did not increase the minute volume, but that the minute volume fell almost in the same ratio as the pulse increased—so inefficient did the heart become.

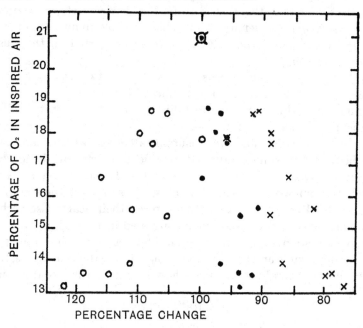

- ● BLOOD FLOW
- ✗ SYSTOLIC OUTPUT
- ○ PULSE RATE

Fig. 43.

	Attack (1)	Attack (2)	After attack (1)	Norma
Pulse rate	175	198	82	64
Minute volume (litres) ...	2·8	2·5	6·1	5·0
Systolic output (c.c.)... ...	16·5	12·9	75	77·5

That the brunt of this disease in the minute volume was borne by the skin is shown by the analysis of a sample of blood taken from one of the cutaneous veins in the arm which was almost completely deprived of its oxygen, whilst the mixed venous blood reaching the

B   9 heart was even in the attack about 40 per cent. saturated instead of about 55 per cent. (the usual figure for the subject). Needless to say, he was deeply cyanosed. The stagnation observed in the cutaneous areas supplies to my mind the answer to a question asked by some of the 1922 Everest party—I think Somervell himself. It was this: "Why was it then after our return to camp, when we commenced breathing oxygen we immediately experienced a sensation of warmth in the skin." I take the answer to be that their hearts, immediately on receiving well oxygenated blood, became able to put out a normal minute volume, and that the skin vessels reverted to their usual condition of tone.

As I write the closing words of this chapter two visions come up before me, one a vision of the memory, the other a vision of the imagination. I think of a comfortable bed-room in Trinity College, Cambridge, the subject of our research on tachycardia, having found exercise "impossible" and life "insupportable" elsewhere, has crawled into bed, and in spite of all that outside comforts can do to warm him he lies there with his skin cyanosed and cold. Then my mind travels to somewhere within a thousand or so feet of the summit of Everest and I conjure up two other figures, their hearts also perhaps beating at 200 a minute, the blood congealed in their skins, but in a place where stagnation means inevitable frost bite, they too found exercise impossible and life insupportable—but in their cases alas, these phases bore a literal significance—how literal all the world knows.

BIBLIOGRAPHY

(1) Fick. *Verh. d. physik. Med. Ges. in Wurtzburg.* Sitziber. 1870, xvi, II. 1872.

(2) Barcroft, Boycott, Dunn and Peters. *Quart. Journ. of Med.* XIII. 35. 1919.

(3) Redfield, Bock and Meakins. *Journ. Physiol.* LVII. 76. 1922.

(4) Christiansen, Douglas and Haldane. *Journ. Physiol.* XLVIII. 262. 1914.

(5) Barcroft and Marshall. *Journ. Physiol.* LVIII. 148. 1923.

(6) Douglas and Haldane. *Journ. Physiol.* LVI. 69. 1922.

(7) Krogh. *Skand. Archiv.* XXVII. 125. 1912.

(8) Starling and Markwalder. *Journ. Physiol.* XLVII. 275. 1913.

(9) Barcroft. *Royal Army Medical Corps Journal,* x. Jan. 1921.

(10) Doi. *Journ. Physiol.* LV. 43. 1921.

(11) Meakins and Davies. *Heart,* IX. 192. 1922.

(12) Stewart, G. N. *Heart,* III. 33. 1911.

(13) Schneider. *Physiol. Reviews,* I. 655. 1921.

(14) Haldane, Kellas and Kennaway. *Journ. Physiol.* LIII. 183. 1919.

(15) Barcroft, Bock and Roughton. *Heart,* IX. 7. 1921.

CHAPTER X

THE STRAIN ON THE HEART

HAVING established the fact that the response of the pulse to exercise—even the ordinary exercise of a rather sedentary existence—is greater at Cerro than at the sea-level, the question naturally arises, how much extra strain is being put upon the heart? The answer to this question is of extreme interest to the physiologist because it involves some sort of definition of what is meant by putting a strain on the heart. It is easy to use a phrase, but to express that phrase in measurements and numbers one must settle just what is to be measured.

Put the question as follows, "What degree of extra effort does the heart undertake" at Cerro de Pasco? I avoid saying "how much extra work does the heart do" because if I put the question in that way, I commit myself to answering it in a certain way. The calculation of the "work done by the heart" is given in every text-book of physiology, and clearly one way of answering the question is to make that calculation and that we may do forthwith.

The same is done in the following way. You conceive of the heart putting out a certain volume of blood at each beat, and putting it out against a certain pressure. This pressure may be visualised as that which would be exerted by a column of blood 160 cm. in height. So far as our measurements went, the arterial pressure and therefore height of the column was approximately the same at Cerro as at the sea-level. The amount of work done by the left ventricle at a beat is the same as if the quantity of blood expelled at each beat was lifted 160 cm. or 1·6 metres in height. To obtain a measure of this work one must multiply the weight of blood by the height it is lifted; we do not yet know the weight of blood put out per beat. It was as follows. Using the figures I put before you in Chapter IX for the blood which flows round the body per minute as measured by the method of triple extrapolation, and combining them with the pulse rate obtained simultaneously, we get the output of the left ventricle per beat:

	Place	Mean minute volume at rest (litres)	Mean pulse rate	Systolic output	
				c.c.	grammes
Meakins	Sea-level	5·2	69	75	79
	Cerro	4·7	81	58	62
Redfield	Sea-level	5·1	60	85	90
	Cerro	4·1	78	53	57

Multiplying the systolic output by the blood pressure we obtain:

		Systolic output grammes	Pressure[1] in metres of blood, say	Mean work in kilogramme metres	Work per min. in kilogramme metres
Meakins	Sea-level	79	1·6	·126	8·8
	Cerro	62	1·6	·099	8·0
Redfield	Sea-level	90	1·6	·144	8·6
	Cerro	57	1·6	·091	7·1

At each beat therefore the left ventricle does only about three-quarters of the work at Cerro that it does at the sea-level. To obtain the work per minute one must multiply the work per beat by the pulse rate, and accordingly the calculation given about it comes out to be slightly less at Cerro than at the sea-level. Of course, if the blood pressure is constant the ratios are simply those of the minute volumes.

But if the heart is doing less work can we regard it as taking a rest? There may obviously be a great difference between what the heart accomplishes and the effort which it puts forth in the doing of it. We must seek some other method for calculating the effort. Let us take the metabolism of the heart as the index of the effort which it is putting forth. Let us then inquire whether the metabolism of the heart can be correlated to any measurements which we possess.

The factors which govern the heart's oxygen intake have been studied in several laboratories. Here I shall only allude to the mammalian heart which has formed the subject of research in Heidelberg by Rohde[1] and at University College, London, by Evans[2]. Granting that the excised heart can be made to beat in a normal, regular and efficient manner, Rohde had in front of him the possibility of estimating the oxygen which the heart was using and at the same time analysing the factors which its activity revealed.

The metabolism depends not at all on the quantity of blood which the heart puts out but on the tension set up in its effort to contract irrespective of whether that effort is successful or the reverse.

In a very beautiful series of researches Rohde came to the following very simple conclusion. The amount of oxygen which the heart uses varies directly in proportion to (1) the rate of the pulse, and (2) the greatest pressure which it sets up at any time, i.e., the systolic pressure.

[1] The systolic pressures for the members of the 1924 Everest Expedition are given by Major Hingston. The obvious point which they show is a considerable drop of pressure as the subject rises from 16,500 to 21,000 feet. Possibly, but not certainly, there is a maximal value between 7000 and 16,000 feet.

If Q be the quantity of oxygen used per minute, T the tension set up and R the rate of the pulse, then

$$\frac{Q}{RT} = \text{a constant.}$$

Evans also found that when the pulse was quickened by rise of temperature the metabolism of the heart varied with the pulse rate.

Let us look back now to the example which was given above of Prof. Meakins's pulse. Let us assume, as was approximately the case, that the blood pressure was the same both at Cerro and at the sea-level—then instead of writing

Effort (= metabolism), varies as pressure × pulse rate,

we can write

Effort (= metabolism), varies as pulse rate.

The pulse rate at sea-level is 69 resting.

  ,,   ,,   Cerro ,, 81 ,,

So that the difference in effort is increased 20 per cent. or thereabouts, whilst the actual work accomplished per minute was diminished by 10 per cent. It would seem that the heart at Cerro was working less economically than at the sea-level.

If we go no further than Rohde and Evans's views, and if the blood pressure remains constant, we may take the minute volume as being the measure of what is accomplished and the pulse rate as the measure of the effort put forth to accomplish it, in which case

$$\frac{\text{min. vol.}}{\text{pulse rate}} = \text{systolic output} = \text{the measure of the heart's efficiency.}$$

But other considerations come in. A series of researches by A. V. Hill[3] on muscle, and Starling[4] and his pupils on the heart—researches which it would be a mere impertinence on my part to call brilliant—have led us to suppose that the measure of the heart's effort at each beat is the extension of the ventricle in diastole. Rohde's view would then only be true subject to the condition that extension in diastole was the same at each beat. Here again we brought home a little scrappy information, enough perhaps to enable us to state the factors concerned in the problem but not much more. Such information as we have comes from the X-ray photographs.

Fig. 44 shows the outlines of the cardiac shadow of Meakins's heart at Cerro (B) and in Edinburgh (A). It is evident that the shadow at Cerro is the smaller of the two, in the absence of any information which would suggest that the back to front diameter increased, we may suppose that the decrease in the area of the shadow, means a decrease in the size of the ventricle. I am far from being an authority on the interpretation of X-ray photographs of the heart, and I found authorities to hold different opinions as to whether the shadow represents the systole or the diastole or either, but fortunately it does not much matter for our present purpose, as the following argument shows. If the shadow represents the systole, we have the information

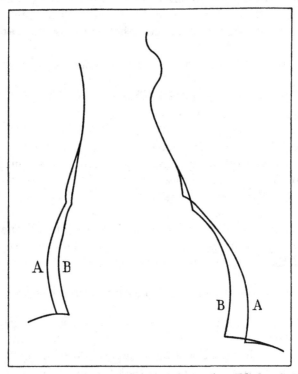

Fig. 44. Outline of shadow of Prof. Meakins's heart, A at Edinburgh, B at Cerro.

that the heart in systole is smaller in volume than at Edinburgh. Now the volume of the ventricle in diastole is equal to that of the ventricle in systole plus the volume of the systolic output. We have already given figures which show that, according to the method of triple extrapolation, the systolic output is smaller at Cerro than at Edinburgh and, according to Meakins's and Davies's method, the systolic output is at least not larger. Therefore on any showing, if the shadow represents the systolic volume it secures us the information that diastolic volume was smaller at Cerro than at sea-level. If this shadow represents the diastolic volume the same is the case. The X-ray shadows of Redfield's and Forbes's hearts told exactly the same story. In the case of Bock and myself it was otherwise, our "shadows did not grow less," unfortunately, but on the other hand they did not increase in size. It would appear that the X-ray shadow divided the hearts into two groups, in one of which the diastolic stretching of the fibres was certainly less at Cerro than at the sea-level, in the other of which it was probably about the same.

In the first group the increase of the pulse rate may not necessarily be a signal of distress, or perhaps I should say that the signal was there but the distress had not yet arrived, for the increased transformation of energy in the cardiac muscle occasioned by the extra beats may have been counterbalanced by the decreased transformation at each beat occasioned by the diminished diastolic stretching of the fibres.

In the second group there was not only the signal but also some small degree of distress. Most likely the alteration in systolic output represented pretty accurately the alteration in the efficiency of the heart's working.

It is of course certain that Bock and I were more affected by the altitude than Meakins, Redfield and Forbes.

The lesson which I think we brought home from Cerro is that in a very fit person with a *very* fit heart there is no strain at 14,000 feet while sitting in a chair, and in a fit person with a fit heart there is not much strain, but here the lesson ends. I must speak a word of warning. The signal of the more rapid pulse has been flown and it behoves the subject to proceed with such caution as the signal may demand. The reader must by no means suppose that I think lightly, on the basis of what I have said above, of the chance of even a fit person straining his heart at high altitudes, and, of course, the data which I have put before him, tell him nothing about an unfit heart. For all we know to the contrary there are hearts which might dilate to a considerable extent at Cerro, as indeed we rather expected ours to do.

One reason for this expectation was the known fact that anoxæmia does cause the heart to dilate. Any person, outside Great Britain, may convince himself of this fact by opening the chest of a cat under urethane (the cat of course receiving artificial respiration), and then watching the heart while gradually cutting down the percentage of oxygen in the air which the cat breathes. The demonstration is a very striking one. I am indebted to Dr Takaeuchi for Fig. 45, which shows the approximate area of the ventral aspect of the cat's heart when its lungs are ventilated: *a*, with oxygen; *b*, rather inefficiently with air; and *c*, with nitrogen in which there is 10 mm. O_2 pressure, the latter of course only for a few minutes. The figures were obtained by placing a glass plate[1] over the heart and drawing on it the outline of the heart as seen through the glass. The records were made permanent by using the glass as a negative and printing from it.

It therefore seems certain that one has only to push the anoxæmia far enough in order to dilate the heart to an extent which is unnatural for the amount of exercise that is being undertaken. The anoxæmia

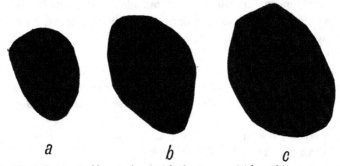

a   *b*   *c*

FIG. 45. Ventral aspect of heart of cat with chest open: (*a*) breathing oxygen; (*b*) air, respiration rather deficient; (*c*) nitrogen containing 10 mm. oxygen pressure.

may be pushed in either one of two ways: (1) by going to a higher level[2], and (2) by taking enough exercise at Cerro.

It is theoretically to be expected (see Chapter v) on the diffusion theory that increased exercise, i.e., increased oxygen absorption by the body, will increase the disparity between the oxygen pressure in the alveolar air and that in the arterial blood. At normal barometric pressures the pressure of oxygen in the alveoli is so high that the pressure of the oxygen in the arterial blood might fall short during exercise by many millimetres of that in the alveolar air, without the arterial blood being sensibly less oxygenated than is normally the case, but at Cerro it is otherwise, any want of equilibrium translates itself at once into a deficiency in saturation and the arterial blood darkens in colour. Here one does not go black in the face when one

[1] More exact records have since been obtained with the cinematograph.

[2] Such a dilatation does take place at higher altitudes. Somervell writes: "All who had gone over 27,000 feet were found by Major Hingston, I.M.S., the Expedition's official doctor, to have dilated hearts, which took one to three weeks to recover."

takes 190 kilometres per minute of exercise on a bicycle ergometer. At Cerro Meakins did, and the colour of his face was a fair index of the saturation of his arterial blood. Before the exercise his arterial saturation was 91 per cent., when he was on the bicycle it went down to 78 per cent. His radial pulse was uncountable. One would like to have had an X-ray shadow of his chest under these circumstances, for it is to be expected that the heart would undergo a degree of dilation on exercise at high altitudes that it does not undergo at low ones. Exercise at Cerro then entails a double strain on the heart, (*a*) because more beats are required for a given piece of work, and (*b*) because the heart is more dilated as the result of exercise and therefore the fibres more stretched.

Here again one's mind reverts to Somervell's statement which I have quoted already. If the strain varies directly with the product of the number of beats and the degree of dilatation, what it must have been when the pulse was more rapid than in the severest exercise, and the dilatation such as might be produced by the great degree of anoxæmia of which man is capable.

BIBLIOGRAPHY

(1) ROHDE. *Arch. f. Exp. Path. and Pharmacol.* LXVIII. 401. 1912.

(2) EVANS, C. L. *Journ. Physiol.* XLV. 213. 1912.

(3) HILL, A. V. *Journ. Physiol.* XLVI. 435. 1913.

(4) PATTERSON, PIPER AND STARLING. *Journ. Physiol.* XLVIII. 465. 1914.

CHAPTER XI

THE NUMBER AND NATURE OF THE RED CORPUSCLES

Of the questions put to me since my return from Peru, perhaps the most frequent has been, Did you obtain an increase in the red cell count? And this seems a little surprising, for I had supposed the question to have been answered in the last century beyond any possibility of doubt. All workers who have made counts at altitudes of above 10,000 feet, and many who have carried out observations at lower levels, have obtained an increase in the number of red cells per cubic millimetre of blood.

A certain topical interest centres around the fact that the increase caused by altitude in the red blood count was discovered in the very locality and at the very altitude at which we worked: "Viault[1] observed the increase in the number of red corpuscles per cubic millimetre in himself and his companions as well as in men and animals resident in the place during a three weeks' visit to a height of 14,400 feet in Peru." Major Hingston[2] obtained quite similar data on the natives of the Pamir Plateau up to 18,200 feet:

Date	Altitude in thousands of feet	Corpuscles millions per cubic mm.
April 10	·7	4·5
May 12	4·4	5·2
May 21	8·0	6·0
May 28	10·0	6·6
May 30	12·0	6·8
June 1	12·4	6·8
June 21	13·3	7·5
June 23	15·6	7·8
June 26	16·9	7·6
July 27	18·2	8·3

In the above table, if x be the increase in the number of corpuscles over the sea-level value, 4·25 millions, and y be the increase in altitude, within the incidental errors of counting etc., $x = ·225y$.

The Pike's Peak party found the same, and as indeed has everyone who has made the test at altitudes which run into five figures. Nor is there any uncertainty about the fact that this increase in red blood corpuscles means an increase in the hæmoglobin value or oxygen capacity of each cubic centimetre of blood. The most elegant demonstration of which is a research carried out by a mining engineer, Mr J. Richards[3] at Dr Haldane's behest. Mr Richards's observations on the hæmoglobin capacity of his own blood at varying altitudes up to about 15,000 feet are given in Fig. 46. The occasion was a journey from Liverpool *via* Buenos Aires to Pazña in Bolivia: "Mr Richards left Liverpool on November 10, reaching Buenos Aires on December 5 and Valparaiso on the 8th after a two days' journey overland. He then sailed up the West Coast to Autofagasta and started thence on the 15th up-country, reaching a height of 12,500 feet on the 17th, and staying at this height till the 24th when he moved to a height of 15,000 feet." Nor is there any doubt that these increases in the red blood count and in the hæmoglobin capacity are in direct response to want of oxygen.

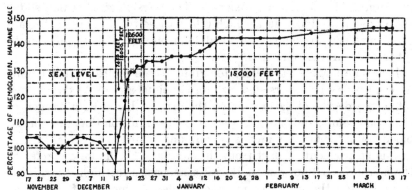

FIG. 46.   .... = Mean percentage of hæmoglobin at sea-level.
────── = Actual percentage determined.

In animals "Jolyet and Sellier found that they could produce polycythæmia by keeping animals in air at normal barometric pressure but deficient in oxygen, while lowering of the barometric pressure proved ineffective so long as the oxygen pressure was kept high." In my "glass case"[4] experiment the parallel observation was made on the oxygen capacity of each cubic millimetre of my blood. It rose from ·180 to ·200 c.c. owing to the "exhibition" (as the pharmacological phrase goes) of my person to an oxygen pressure which fell over six days to a minimum of 87 mm. whilst the total barometric pressure during the period was that of the outside atmosphere, the temperature was normal and the air moist. Seeing that the facts are so well established, why should the medical world have been so curious as to our findings? There is a reason for most things, and before we dismiss the matter on some such arrogant plea as that the medical profession is in its knowledge twenty years behind the facts as known to the physiologist, let us pause to consider whether the last word has really been said. The physiologist is at an advantage in that he can choose his material, all normal persons, and he can choose the altitude at which he desires to work. The doctor must derive his information from a study of men as they come, mostly sick men, and at altitudes which if they can be selected at all, must be chosen because they are beneficial to his patients. What then is to be said if at some health resort, as Switzerland, at an altitude of 5000 or 6000 feet, the doctor obtains the most divergent results upon the blood counts? Well, the basal principle is not that the red blood count is a function of the altitude, but that it is a function of the degree of anoxæmia. The physiologist has not, so far as I know, placed any data which relate these two factors in the case of normal persons who have lived long enough on any altitude to settle to a chronic condition.

I may be forgiven therefore for giving some figures which I hope may some day be superseded by more copious and exact data. They relate the degree of saturation of the arterial blood with oxygen to the blood count, and they start from the assumption that the normal blood count for healthy men is 5·5 millions, whilst the normal saturation is 95 per cent. Apart from the normal (A), the figures refer to three groups: (B) our own party after at least a fortnight's residence at Cerro, (C) the group of mining engineers which staff the place, and (D) the native residents. Groups B and C each contains four persons, group D contains three. The variation between the extremes is:

	Percentage saturation	Blood count, millions
Group B	9	·5
Group C	5·0	·3
Group D	2·7	·2

The results are as shown in Fig. 47.

So far as our meagre data go, the relation between the degree of saturation of the arterial blood and the number of red corpuscles appears to be a very direct one, and much more so than that between the altitude and the blood count. Indeed, it must be borne in mind that even at the sea-level, unsaturation of the arterial blood will produce a polycythæmia of the red cells.

It seems desirable that someone with a genius for the performance of arterial punctures should at some lower altitude compare the unsaturation of the arterial blood with the red count and hæmoglobin value over a considerable series of cases. As I have pointed out elsewhere in this volume, there is no difficulty in accounting for the existence of anoxæmia in persons with unsound lungs, at much lower altitudes than would be the case with subjects blessed with an ideal

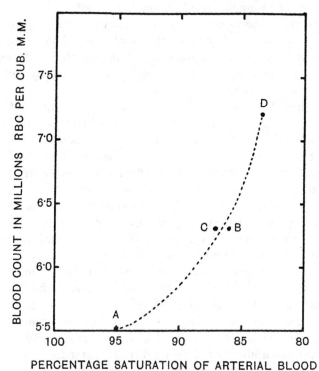

FIG. 47. A, party, sea-level; B, party, Cerro; C, engineers, Cerro; D, natives, Cerro.

pulmonary "outfit." Suppose that some parts of the lung are deficient either in elasticity or in permeability, the deficiency may be great enough to allow of the blood leaving them in an unsaturated condition at 6000 or 7000 feet altitude, yet not great enough to produce any appreciable degree of unsaturation at the normal atmospheric pressure. Such persons never would reach 14,000 feet and to their absence is probably attributable the uniformity of the results obtained on the dwellers at really high altitudes. Yet even now I do not think the doctor's case has been completely stated. For behind this anxiety to know whether the red count had increased, there was, I fancy, a consciousness, or perhaps rather a subconsciousness, of an obscure, an intensely interesting mechanism which as yet is not understood. (1) How does a deficiency of the saturation in the arterial blood produce an increase in the number of red cells, both in each cubic centimetre of blood and in the total quantity of blood in the body? (2) How does such a deficiency produce an increase in the total amount of hæmoglobin which the body contains?

Are these two questions (1) and (2) really the same question, or are the mechanisms which regulate the number of red blood corpuscles and those which regulate the quantity of hæmoglobin quite separate and distinct? These questions cannot be answered fully, but some sort of preliminary analysis is worth while.

Firstly, then, how do we know that the total quantity of hæmoglobin in the body and the total number of red corpuscles which the blood as a whole contains, are increased by residence at altitudes of 14,000 feet? That point was proven beyond any reasonable doubt by the Pike's Peak [5] Expedition in 1911. The charts (Fig. 48) published in their report make the matter quite clear.

In the discussion of how the increase is brought about, one must recognise at once that there is probably no one method. The body works as a team and several quite different mechanisms may be brought into play, each of which, because it only is asked to contribute a little, suffers no great dislocation of function. These mechanisms may be divided into emergency measures—a sort of first aid—and final measures. Let us consider the emergency measures first.

Of the emergency method for the increase of the number of corpuscles in each cubic millimetre of blood the first which we must consider as a possibility is the abstraction of water from the plasma. This process would not alter the total quantity of hæmoglobin in circulation and of course it would not alter the quantity of hæmoglobin in such corpuscle. The colour index would therefore be unchanged.

The concentration of the blood by reduction of the volume of plasma was first put forward by Abderhalden [6] on the basis of experiments carried out on two series of rabbits, one killed at Basle, the other at San Mauritz. The latter were found to have no more hæmoglobin in circulation—per animal, not per kilo of animal—than the former, though this had a higher blood count. The rabbits killed at San Mauritz had a higher hæmoglobin content per kilo, than those killed at Basle, but that was due to the fact that they lost weight.

The view that the blood loses water when the organism is exposed to a low oxygen pressure is very easy to understand. It is only

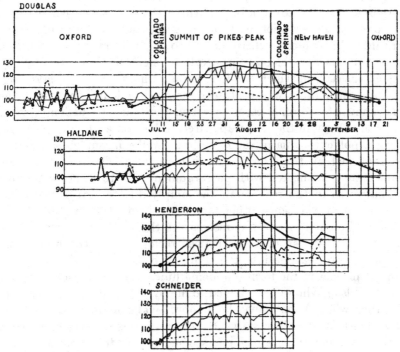

Fig. 48. Abscissæ and ordinates on the same scale in each case. Ordinates represent percentages of average values obtained before the ascent of the Peak (Oxford and Colorado Springs) on the particular subject.

  ——— = percentages of hæmoglobin.
  .... = blood volume.
  ——— = total oxygen capacity or total amount of hæmoglobin.

necessary to suppose that intermediate products of metabolism are formed during the activity of the organs, that these diffuse but slowly from the seat of their formation, that in the meantime they raise the osmotic pressure of the tissues in which they are formed and which in their turn imbibed water from the plasma; or alternatively that under incompletely ærobic conditions products are produced which increase the permeability of the capillaries, such as are found by Dale and Laidlaw[7] to appear during tissue breakdown caused by injury. The difficulty is not that of formulating a theory of the way in which concentration of the blood, due to loss of fluid, might take place but of securing the actual evidence of its occurrence.

During the war the mechanism of blood concentration was much discussed, for a number of conditions occurred in which the red corpuscle count rose rapidly. Of these the one which came under my personal observation was that of gas poisoning with pulmonary irritants. In such cases there seemed to me, as in mountain sickness, to be two phases of blood concentration, one, that shown by recently gassed cases (8), in which the lesion was of hours' or days' standing, and in which there was profuse pulmonary œdema, the other was that shown by chronic cases in which the œdema had long passed away (9). Of these the latter appeared to be "on all fours" with the chronic polycythæmia of the mountain dweller inasmuch as it could be abolished by the administration of oxygen. The former is that immediately connected with our argument. As to whether the immediate rise in the red count was simply due to loss of water, or whether there was some other factor involved, there was some difference of opinion between ourselves and the American workers. The American view was that the concentration of the corpuscles was simply due to leakage into the connective tissue and alveoli of the lung of plasma in the form of œdema fluid. Lieut. Goldschmidt and Lieut. Wilson, who were seconded to me by the American gas service, and than whom I shall never have more loyal colleagues, strove hard to convert me to their view. So far as I was concerned it went entirely against the grain, for it seemed to pay too small a tribute to the water-regulating mechanism of the body. Looking back, I must admit that whichever way the grain of my particular mind runs, the figures are entirely in support of Goldschmidt's and Wilson's contention. Their two principal points were as follows: (1) that the loss of water by the blood never exceeded the volume of the œdema fluid; (2) that the concentration of the blood was uninfluenced by the quantity of oxygen in the atmosphere inhaled—that is to say, that placing the gassed animals in an atmosphere rich in oxygen did not prevent the concentration of blood, as compared with that which took place in control animals gassed to the same extent but inspiring atmospheric air.

If the American view is correct, one cannot hope to support the contention that oxygen want produces an immediate concentration of the blood by producing osmotic changes in the tissues by an appeal to the phenomena of acute phosgene poisoning. One must turn in some other direction. Evidence that want of oxygen can produce some degree of œdema in the one organ, namely, the central nervous system, is adduced by Forbes, Cobb and Fremont-Smith(10), who describe it as following on carbon monoxide poisoning.

So much then for the possibility of concentration by the rapid withdrawal of water. What is there to be said about the complementary possibility—that of the rapid addition of corpuscles to the blood in an emergency?

At this point we may pause for a moment to consider the extent to which the evidence of rapid blood concentration is illusory. Most of it, of course, comes from determinations—blood counts or hæmoglobin determinations—made on blood taken from cutaneous areas. The most usual places for the withdrawal of blood are the finger and the ear. That samples of blood which were obtained from various parts of the cutaneous areas might differ from that obtained from other places was originally demonstrated by Foa(11) and appropriately enough on Monte Rosa, that it is not necessarily so was shown by Dallwig, Kolls and Loewenhart(12). Whilst congestion in the skin is an obvious source of fallacy there seems to be no doubt that the later workers have been quite alive to it. There is therefore every reason to believe that the concentration of red blood corpuscles does take place in the general circulation as well as in the skin.

But to return to the question of whether blood can receive any rapid accession of corpuscles from areas in which they are stored, the considerations which have just been discussed point to one such possibility. If at one time corpuscles can accumulate in the skin, to be returned subsequently to the blood, may there not normally be accumulations of which the blood can avail itself if necessary? The possibilities in this direction are relatively unexplored. It is only necessary to read Prof. Krogh's masterly book on the capillary circulation to appreciate the ease with which corpuscles in considerable numbers might be hidden away in capillaries which were cut off from the general circulation and produced on demand.

There is one organ however to which more than a passing reference must be made in this connection—the spleen. Quite recently a series of researches has shed some new light on the physiology of the spleen. The story commenced on our way to Peru. It had been our intention to measure the total quantity of hæmoglobin in the body during our stay in the mountains. To this end we desired to start from an assured base line, and therefore to make numerous and accurate observations of the oxygen capacity of the blood at sea-level. For this purpose, whenever the weather served we measured the amount of hæmoglobin in our bodies by the carbon monoxide method which seems to be the most satisfactory method for the purpose. These measurements were made on Meakins, Doggart and myself, and in all cases with the same result, namely that the hæmoglobin content of all our bodies appeared to rise day by day, reaching a maximum at the time when we passed through the Panama Canal, and then sinking somewhat, but not to the same extent. The observations were repeated with the same general result, but not quite so clearly cut, on the way home. This additional observation was made, namely that the excess of corpuscles did not appear to be due to the accession of immature forms to the blood. With the very interesting correspondence between the apparent quantity of hæmoglobin in our circulations and the temperature of the region at which the observations were made we are not here concerned, that is a story of its own; here we merely observe that considerable changes in the apparent amount of hæmoglobin in the body can be brought about more suddenly than could be accounted for by the manufacture of fresh pigment of the bone marrow, and consisting of corpuscles which show no sign of being immature. The work was repeated on our return home. Two subjects, Davies and Fetter[13], were put into the respiration chamber which was maintained at a temperature of over 90° F. for three days. In each case the apparent amount of hæmoglobin in the circulation increased, but only on the last day was there any sign of immature cells. It may be of significance that the increase in hæmoglobin value only appeared to take place in the day-time. At night the blood volume increased apparently by mere dilution, reminding one of the results obtained by Barbour and Tolstoi who found an increase in the water content of dogs placed in warm baths, a result which depends[14] upon the integrity of the nervous system. The question then arose, whence came these corpuscles? Here again it is possible—even probable—that some came from capillaries in the skin; that in the warm temperature circulation in the skin was good and the capillaries mostly open, whilst at ordinary temperatures some of the cutaneous capillaries were closed for more than the twenty minutes during which we were breathing carbon monoxide.

In seeking for some storehouse from which corpuscles can be produced on emergency, one's mind naturally turns to those situations in which the red cells are entirely outside the system of arteries, veins and capillaries, of such the most obvious is the spleen. Can the corpuscles in the spleen pulp be regarded as physiologically within the circulation? If not, can they be added to the circulating corpuscles if need be? If the spleen is a storehouse, what stimuli serve to unlock its doors? The answer to the first question is furnished by placing animals in an atmosphere which contains small quantities of carbon monoxide and comparing the relative percentages of carboxy-hæmoglobin in the hæmoglobin of the spleen pulp and in the general circulation. This best shows the spleen pulp, physiologically, to be quite unexpectedly remote from the circulating blood (15), (16). If the animal, a guinea-pig, be in some such concentration of CO as will produce 20 per cent. saturation in his blood, two hours may elapse before any CO can be detected in his spleen pulp at all, and upwards of six hours before the corpuscles in the spleen become 20 per cent. saturated. The answer to the second question is that the spleen can be made to contribute its corpuscles in part to the blood, and to the third that oxygen want, either by reduction of oxygen in the inspired air, or addition of CO to the same, will cause the spleen to contract down and express many of the corpuscles in the pulp into the circulation (17). It is not suggested that oxygen want is the only *sesame*, forms of agitation which cause a secretion of adrenalin will do the same; but oxygen want is the key which is of most account in the present connection. The administration of carbon monoxide, reducing as it does the amount of oxyhæmoglobin in circulation, is the form of stimulus which has been worked out most completely.

A sufficient dose will reduce the spleen to about half its former size. That the material expressed is largely corpuscles is shown by the fact that the blood which flows into the splenic vein when the spleen is contracting contains a markedly less percentage of carboxy-hæmoglobin than does the arterial blood which is entering the organ at the same time. The actual hæmoglobin in the spleen pulp of course contains less than either.

There may be other unexposed situations in which mature corpuscles may be stored and from which they may be produced in emergency, but when the emergency methods have been exhausted the great and final means of augmentation of the hæmoglobin value of the body is increased production of the pigment wrought in the bone marrow. Before we pass to the consideration of the marrow let us tabulate the position so far:

SCHEME 6

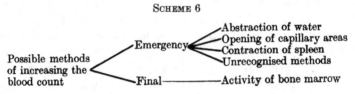

The evidence of increased activity of the bone marrow which was put forward by Zuntz and his colleagues [18] was derived from observation of the venous blood coming from the marrow in animals and also of sections of the marrow itself. The increased activity which they observed was referred by him, no doubt correctly, to the decreased pressure of oxygen in the air, as shown by the work of Dallwig, Kolls and Loewenhart [12].

The desirability of obtaining some quantitative evidence of young corpuscles in the blood at high altitudes led to some very interesting work by Morawitz [19]. The following is a brief account of Morawitz's argument. If blood—even sterile blood—be sealed up in a tube it darkens in colour slowly, the oxyhæmoglobin becoming reduced. The blood, in short, has a certain metabolism of its own of a very low order. It has been measured quantitatively by Douglas [20] and Krogh [21] and its nature investigated by Morawitz. It is not a property of the plasma, and, on the other hand, it is not confined to the white blood corpuscles which, of course, like all other nucleated structures, have quite a considerable metabolism for their size. The red corpuscles have a very low metabolism also. One imagines three sorts of structure in normal blood: (1) the leucocytes which have a high specific coefficient of oxidation, but which are present in so small a bulk that their metabolism is a practically negligible factor in that of the whole blood; (2) the red blood corpuscles which have a very slight specific coefficient of oxidation, but which on account of their large bulk are responsible chiefly for such oxidation as takes place in the blood; and (3) the plasma which has no specific oxidation at all. We will confine ourselves to the consideration of the second category. The next point which Morawitz made was that the degree of respiration of the red corpuscles depended upon their age. If the organism was subjected to any experimental procedure, such as repeated bleedings, which increased the proportion of young red cells in the circulation, the blood reduced itself much more rapidly as the result. For instance healthy rabbits were given daily injections of phenyl hydrazine hydrochloride until they became anæmic. When the hæmoglobin content had reached about 2 per cent. of its former value, blood was withdrawn from the carotid or other artery by means of an aseptic operation, defibrinated by shaking with glass beads and thoroughly shaken with oxygen. One portion of the blood was analysed at once in the Barcroft-Haldane apparatus, the remainder, about 3 c.c., was placed in a glass bottle from which air was excluded, and kept in a water bath at a known temperature for a known time. The oxygen present was then analysed. An example will perhaps make the method more clear.

Rabbit 3. Made anæmic by injections of phenyl-hydrazine between May 10 and June 4. Hæmoglobin value sank to 18 per cent. Bled and killed June 4. Maximal oxygen capacity of 1 c.c. of blood 0·043 c.c. After two hours at room temperature oxygen in blood nil.

The work was continued by Itami [22] who followed the whole course of numerous cases of anæmia produced experimentally both in dogs and rabbits. The anæmia was in some cases from hæmorrhage and in some cases induced by phenyl-hydrazine. The technique was the same as that of Morawitz.

Let us consider some abstracts of typical experiments. The first shows the effect of continuous bleeding. It is evident from the last column but one that as more and more new corpuscles were produced the oxygen consumption of the blood itself became greater and greater in amount, corresponding to the increased number of young corpuscles present.

Rabbit (male), 2900 grams

Number of days after bleeding	Red blood corpuscles, millions	Nucleated elements, thousands	Oxygen capacity	O₂ content after five hours per cent.	O₂ used up in five hours per cent.	Bleeding c.c.
1	5·2	6·5	15·2	14·1	8	20
3	4·8	3·3	13·7	12·1	14	20
5	4·5	4·9	12·6	10·1	21	30
7	4·1	5	12·5	3·8	60	35
9	3·3	6·5	10·0	2·6	75	—

Morawitz [23] transferred the argument to high altitudes and concluded that if residence at 10,000 feet caused an increased production of corpuscles the blood withdrawn at these altitudes would reduce itself more rapidly than that withdrawn at sea-level. The following table shows that at Col d'Olen he obtained no evidence of increased blood formation and only a trifling rise in the red blood count.

Subject of research, E. M.

Date	Hb value of blood	No. of red corpuscles in millions per cub. mm.	Oxygen capacity in vols. per cent.		O_2 diminution vols. per cent.	Place
			Freshly shaken	After five hours' incubation		
July 28	108	5·3	20·4	19·5	0·9	} Heidelberg
31	113	—	20·7	20·2	0·5	
Aug. 12	112	5·5				
13–17	—	—	—	—	—	Small journeys
19	—	—	—	—	—	Climb to Col d'Olen
22	117	6·0	22·3	21·5	0·8	
23	—	5·8	—	—	—	} Col d'Olen,
25	118	6·1	21·8	21·2	0·6	3000 m.
27	122	5·3	23·0	22·0	0·8	

So much for the results obtained by Morawitz and his pupil Itami. Let us now turn to another test for young red corpuscles, namely the presence of "reticulated red cells."

When human blood is stained with cresyl blue the great majority of the red blood corpuscles do not stain, but there are always a few containing a reticulum which show the blue stain. Normally they form about one to one-and-a-half per cent. of the erythrocytes, but in certain affections there is a measurable, and in others there is a considerable, increase in the number of reticulated cells present. Such diseases are those in which loss, and consequent formation of blood cells, take place. It is generally held that the reticulated cells are cells which emerge at an unusually early age from the bone marrow. The reticulated cell then is a young red corpuscle; normally it spends its life in the marrow until very shortly before the reticulum disappears[24]. As we have indicated above, a cubic millimetre of blood usually contains about 50,000 such.

We have alluded to the presence of reticulated cells as "another test" contrasting it with that previously discussed, namely the power of the blood to reduce itself. In reality the contrast is of the most superficial nature, for Harrop[24], one of my own party in Peru, showed that the percentage of reticulated cells and the reducing character of the blood went hand-in-hand, the suggestion being that it is the reticulated cells which by their relatively high metabolism

are principally responsible for the power of the blood to convert its
own oxygen into carbonic acid. The character of Harrop's evidence
appears in the following table:

Oxygen consumed in six hours' incubation in volumes per 100 of blood	Percentage of reticulated cells	Condition
1	0·5–1	Normal
1·3	2	Carcinoma of stomach
1·22	2·3	Pernicious anæmia
1·56	3–4	Hodgkin's disease
3·25	12 ⎫	Congenital hæmolytic
4·44	13·1 ⎭	jaundice

Both tests, then, may be and have been used to indicate blood
formation, the general argument being that both tests indicate young
and live cells, and that these are a sign of intensive formation of
erythrocytes. Such at all events was our idea in testing for reticulated
cells in Peru. It was known that the number of red cells and the
amount of hæmoglobin in the body increased. Were these increases
due to diminished destruction or to increased production? This
could be tested perhaps by the viability of the blood, and of this
viability we chose the reticulated cells as the criterion.

A good example of the changes which took place in the various
members of the party is shown in Fig. 49.

The following features of the graph should be made clear:

(1) That Dr Bock's blood started with a constant level of reticulated
cells at or close to the normal figure.

(2) That with a slight lag the number of cells rises abruptly and
remains much increased during the whole of our stay on "the Hill."

(3) That it descended, and for some time after we reached the sea
level was markedly below the normal level.

If there was nothing more to be said than what has appeared so
far in the discussion, the conclusion would be that on ascending there
is a considerable formation of new cells, that this formation continued
while we were at Cerro de Pasco, and that it stopped when we came
down, and indeed the output became much smaller than is normally
the case. The data, however, which are shown in Fig. 50 made us
pause before drawing any such conclusion.

Fig. 50 shows the number of reticulated cells not only in our own
bloods but in those of the engineers and of the native population.
In each case the reticulated count is increased and nearly to the same

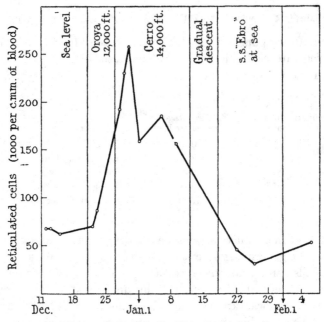

FIG. 49. Reticulated cells in Bock's blood

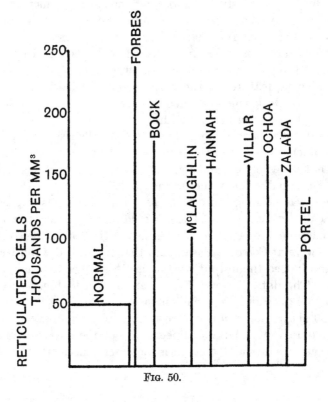

FIG. 50.

extent. Are we then to draw the inference that men whose parents and grandparents have been in the mountains are still making and destroying corpuscles to an extent which can only be matched at the sea-level by such a case as one of pernicious anæmia? Of course it is possible that such might be the case, that to keep their red cell count up to 7–8 millions they still had recourse to this riot of blood formation and destruction. Fortunately I had the help of Dr Cecil Dinker of Harvard Medical School in the interpretation of this diagram. In the light of the information which he gave me a much more simple explanation appeared possible, making but two assumptions: (1) that the red blood corpuscle at Cerro has a life-time of the same length as at sea-level; (2) that a given quantity of the red marrow in the bones produces corpuscles at the same rate there as here.

It will be clear that if the number of corpuscles in the blood increases from 5,000,000 to 7,500,000 per cubic mm., i.e., a 50 per cent. increase, the amount of marrow must increase in the same ratio. The cavity in the bones, however, which contains the marrow remains the same size. This cavity is a good deal larger than the marrow under normal circumstances. The remainder of the cavity is filled largely by fat, but to some extent by the store of maturing reticulated cells, which as they grow older are gradually becoming less reticulated until they are ready to merge into the general circulation. To make room for the new marrow this store must be scrapped and the reticulated cells thrust sooner from within their bony hiding place into the peripheral vessels. Time has not increased the cavities in the "Cholos" bones, nor has it diminished the amount of marrow necessary to manufacture a given quantity of corpuscles. Hence the reticulated cells are still extruded at an early stage, but probably not in greater numbers than corresponds to the increase in the number of red blood corpuscles.

Till quite recently no question has been raised but that the increase of red blood corpuscles was the direct result of the fall in barometric pressure and most observers have attributed it to the decrease of oxygen pressure in the blood. Within the last few years quite a new theory has been put forward by Kestner[25] who "considers that the effective factor of high climate is not diminished oxygen content but the increased and more intense irradiation by the sun's rays. By the effect of rays substances are formed in the air which stimulate the formation of red blood corpuscles if they (the rays) are inhaled. It is possible that these unknown substances are nitroxyl compounds. If the irradiated air is conducted through a solution of potassium iodide starch in the dark an intense blue colour appears"[26]. The above conclusion was based on experiments made upon dogs.

Without further research it is not possible to state the precise amount of weight to give to Kestner's experiments. That a low oxygen pressure in the atmosphere does lead to an increase in the hæmoglobin value of the blood was shown in "the glass case experiment" in which in six days the hæmoglobin value of my blood rose from 95 to 105. While Kestner's view may not represent the whole truth it may still constitute a very real part of it. That it should have been put forward by a physiologist of such high standing forms a very pertinent answer to a question put to me shortly before I went to Peru by a very great authority: "Why go to the Andes to study high altitudes when you can do it all in your chamber"?

BIBLIOGRAPHY

(1) VIAULT. *Comptes Rendus*, III. 91, 1890.

(2) HINGSTON. *Indian Journal of Medical Research*, IX. 173. 1921.

(3) RICHARDS. *Phil. Trans.* B. CCIII. 316, Appendix I. 1913.

(4) BARCROFT, COOKE, HARTRIDGE, PARSONS AND PARSONS. *Journ. Physiol.* LIII. CX. 1920.

(5) DOUGLAS, HALDANE, HENDERSON AND SCHNEIDER. *Phil. Trans. Roy. Soc.* B. CCIII. 299. 1913.

(6) ABDERHALDEN. *Zeitsch. f. Physiol. Chem.* XXII. 526. 1896-7.

(7) DALE AND LAIDLAW. *Journ. Physiol.* LII. 355. 1919.

(8) DUFTON. *Chemical Warfare Medical Committee Report*, No. IV. 4.

(9) BARCROFT, DUFTON AND HUNT. *Quart. Journal of Medicine*, XIII. 179. 1920.

(10) FORBES, COBB AND FREMONT-SMITH. *Archives of Neurology and Psychiatry*, II. 264. 1924.

(11) FOA. *Laboratoire Scientifique International du Mont Rosa.* Turin, 1904.

(12) DALLWIG, KOLLS AND LOEWENHART. *Amer. Journ. Physiol.* XXXIX. 77. 1915.

(13) BARCROFT, DAVIES, FETTER AND SCOTT. *Phil. Trans.* B. CCXI. 455. 1923.

(14) BARBOUR AND TOLSTOI. *American Journ. Physiol.* LIX. Proc. 488. 1922.

(15) BARCROFT, J. AND H. *Journ. Physiol.* LVIII. 138. 1923.

(16) HANAK AND HARKAVY. *Journ. Physiol.* LIX. 121. 1924.

(17) DE BOER AND CARROLL. *Journ. Physiol.* LIX. 312. 1924.

(18) ZUNTZ, LOEWY, MÜLLER AND CASPARI. *Hohenklima und Bergwanderungen*, p. 186. Berlin, 1906.

(19) MORAWITZ. *Archiv. für. Exp. Path. und Pharm.* LX. 298. 1909.

(20) DOUGLAS. *Journ. Physiol.* XXXIX. 453. 1910.

(21) KROGH. *Skand. Arch.* XXIII. 193. 1910.

(22) ITAMI UND MORAWITZ. *Deutsch. Archiv. f. Klin. Med.* C. 191. 1910.

(23) MORAWITZ UND MASIG. *Deutsch. Med. Wochenschr.* Nr. 8. 1910.

(24) HARROP. *Arch. Int. Med.* XXIII. 745. 1919.

(25) KESTNER. *Zeitsch. f. Biol.* LXXIII. 1. 1921.

(26) WASTL. *Physiol. Abstr.* CXXX. 1921.

CHAPTER XII

THE MIND

In Schneider's article [1] I observed the following words: "Barcroft has pointed out that acute want of oxygen simulates drunkenness, while chronic anoxæmia, which is an oxygen want (perhaps not very great, but which may be continued over months), simulates fatigue." I had forgotten that I had expressed myself quite so definitely as this, but the statement is not seriously in error. At all events, we may examine the effects of oxygen want from just this point of view. To what extent does acute oxygen want simulate drunkenness? Oxygen want may be so acute as to be quickly fatal. In that case it cannot be said that it offers any real analogy to drunkenness. The following, for instance, has taken place. A man has been re-breathing a relatively small quantity of air from a rubber bag. The air passes over alkali, so that the carbonic acid is all absorbed, the air, however, is constantly becoming poorer in oxygen as his system absorbs that gas. The man gets darker and darker in colour, and finally, and perhaps without much warning, drops on the floor.

I have seen animals pass out in much the same way, i.e., a rabbit which had been gassed with phosgene the day previously, and which was suffering from pneumonia to the point of being cyanosed, was placed in a waste paper basket some ten inches deep. It leaped out of the basket, but as the result of the effort it collapsed on the floor and died immediately. It may here be explained that whilst the amount of muscular contraction which would be involved in the leap would not appreciably affect the oxygen content in the arterial blood of a normal rabbit, the same amount of exercise considerably reduces the oxygen content of the arterial blood in an animal which is already anoxic. There were cases also in the war where apparently the trouble was want of oxygen brought about by exposure to pulmonary irritants, in which death on exertion was quite sudden.

Passing to cases somewhat less extreme, however, we come to those in which the experimenter is placed in a chamber in which the oxygen pressure is reduced and observations made on his mental condition. Into this category would come also some cases which have been observed on balloon ascents.

In these cases unconsciousness is the final result—as in extreme cases of alcoholic excess—but before that condition is reached stages of mental abnormality are passed through which are certainly rather like those of drunkenness.

Two instances, both contributed to the literature by Dr Haldane, may be referred to. I place them side by side here because they illustrate incidentally the similarity of symptoms produced in two quite different kinds of anoxæmia.

The first to which I shall refer is an account given by the late Sir Clement le Neve Foster (2) of experiences which he suffered during an investigation of the causes of one of the most tragic mining catastrophes in the British Isles. The accident was in the Isle of Man in the year 1897. Dr le Neve Foster was the Chief Government Inspector of Mines in Great Britain, and, having gone down the mine after the accident, he became the victim of carbon monoxide poisoning. The carbon monoxide, so far as is known, has no direct effect upon the system, but it monopolises the hæmoglobin of the blood corpuscles, preventing the carriage of oxygen to the brain and other tissues. The anoxæmia of carbon monoxide poisoning is therefore an example of what I have termed the anæmic variety.

The following is the account of Sir Clement le Neve Foster's experiences, as written in his note-book:

How soon I realised that we were in what is commonly called "a tight place" I cannot say; but eventually, from long force of habit, I presume, I took out my note-book. At what o'clock I first began to write I do not know, for the few words written on the first page have no hour put to them. They were simply a few words of good-bye to my family, badly scribbled. The next page is headed "2 A.M.," and I perfectly well recollect taking out my watch from time to time. As a rule I do not take a watch underground but I carried it on this occasion in order to be sure that I left the rat long enough when testing with it. In fact, my note on the day of our misadventure was: "5th ladder. Rat two minutes at man," meaning by the side of the corpse. My notes at 2 P.M. were as follows: "2 P.M. good-bye, we are all dying, your Clement, I fear we are all dying, good-bye, all my darlings all, no help coming, good-bye we are dying, good-bye, good-bye we are dying, no help comes, good-bye, good-bye." Then later, partly scribbled over some "good-byes," I find: "we saw body at 130 and then all became affected by the bad air, we have got to the 115 and can go no further, the box does not come in spite of our ringing for help. It does not come, does not come. I wish the box would come. Captain R. is shouting, my legs are bad, and I feel very...[1], my knees are...[1]." The so-called "ringing" was signalling to the surface by striking the air-pipe with a hammer or bar of iron. We had agreed upon signals before we went down. There is writing over other writing, as if I did not see exactly where I placed my pencil, and then: "I feel as if I was dreaming, no real pain, good-bye, good-bye, I feel as if I were sleeping." "2.15, we are all done. No...[1], or scarcely any, we are done, we are done, gods bye my darlings." Here it is rather interesting to note the "gods" instead of "good."
Before very long the fresh men who had climbed down to rescue us seem to have arrived, and explained that the "box" was caught in the shaft. Judging by my notes I did not realise thoroughly that we should be rescued. Among them occur,

---

[1] Writing became illegible at this point.

"No pain, it is merely like a dream, no pain; no pain, for the benefit of others I say no pain at all, no pain, no pain," I frequently wrote the same sentence over and over again. My last note on reaching the surface tells of that resistance to authority which likewise appears to be a symptom of the poisoning.

Two points I should like particularly to emphasise. First, the constant repetition cannot pass unnoticed; the second is perhaps not very obvious in the extract given but was stressed in the account as I have heard it in conversation, namely, that although Foster knew that he had only a short way to go in order to reach a place of safety, he persisted in sitting where he was, and repeating "Good-bye my darlings, good-bye, good-bye." He seemed unable to follow up the knowledge of what to do by the trifling degree of initiative necessary to carry it into action. As I think of le Neve Foster sitting there saying his "good-byes" when all he had to do was to get up and walk away, I cannot help recollecting that while some of our party suffered more or less from mountain sickness either at Oroya or at Cerro, it occurred to no single one of us to try whether oxygen, which was available enough, would bring relief.

The second example of acute anoxæmia was carried out by Dr Haldane, Dr Kellas, Mr J. B. S. Haldane and Dr Kennaway [3] in the steel chamber at the Brompton Chest Hospital in London. Dr Haldane and Dr Kellas were put in the chamber, air was pumped out, the barometer falling gradually in consequence.

I will pass over the observations up to the point at which Dr Haldane's mental faculties appeared to become impaired. That point corresponded to a barometric pressure of 320 mm. (24,500 feet). Here he had great difficulty in making observations, especially in calculating the pulse rate from 20-second observations and in remembering the position of the second-hand of the watch, at which the observations commenced at 300 mm. pressure. Haldane's reply to all questions with regard to the regulation of the pressure was "keep it at 320." Persons outside were impatient and anxious, and put up messages at the window of the chamber, but Kellas only smiled and referred to Haldane who invariably gave the old answer, "Keep it at 320." Now comes one of the most interesting observations, the pressure was allowed to rise to 350. Haldane's faculties commenced to return. He took up a mirror to examine the colour of his lips and for some little time he endeavoured to carry out this observation with the wrong side of the mirror. Altogether Haldane and Kellas were at 320 mm. or less for an hour; after coming out Haldane was quite unconscious of the lapse of time so spent.

A curious enough experiment this, two men of scientific eminence, one now dead in the pursuit of his goal, shut in a chamber with their friends looking in through the window. The mental faculties of each were so crippled that neither would stop the experiment. Haldane conscious but unable to make scientific observations and repeating the phrase "Keep it at 320," though the barometric pressure had already sunk many millimetres below that point. Kellas grinning through the glass and writing down everything, but unable to appreciate that the man from whom he was taking orders was incoherent, and failing to do other than continue the routine observations on an experiment which has already gone too far.

When these observations had ended two others went into the chamber, the pressure was reduced to 330 mm. and in time those outside, getting uneasy, let in some air. This act of solicitude prompted an expression of resentment on the part of one of those inside which was couched in language so far removed from anything that would be possible in ordinary life as to indicate that control of self and knowledge of "the fitness of things" had vanished as completely as if the experimenter were under the influence of alcohol. Indeed, he wrote shortly before the end of the experiment, "like last stages of drunk. Respirations 45. Pulse can't take."

A while ago during some experiments on the measurement of the rate of flow of blood round the body some information turned up which was of interest as showing that in acute anoxic anoxæmia as in drunkenness the highest faculties are those which disappear first. The routine consisted of expiring all possible air from the lungs, breathing in nitrogen, holding the breath a certain time and then blowing it out in a particular way. The "particular way" involved the turning of certain taps in a Haldane gas analysis apparatus in a given order. The routine was quite simple when I was at rest. Holding the breath for any time up to half a minute with the lungs full of nitrogen, I could collect the sample of expired air without error, or at least generally without error. When exercise was being taken and therefore the degree of anoxæmia was more acute, the routine broke down. The point of particular interest was the precise way in which my faculties fell short of what was required of them. They were unable to think out, or initiate the various steps of the routine. I would sit impotently before the Haldane apparatus when the time arrived for taking the sample. It was not that I was unable to carry out the operations: if I was told what to do I could respond perfectly. Each step in the routine, the turning of the taps, the blowing out of the alveolar air, etc., could be done in order, if a clear command were given of what to do at each point, so that every action was reduced to an elaborate reflex.

Incidentally another observation was made in these experiments which is worth recording though it has little to do with the simulation of drunkenness. When the anoxæmia reached a certain stage my left wrist, which had been motionless with the forearm horizontal, fell into an involuntary rhythm, my hand moving upwards and downwards more or less after the fashion familiar to those of a previous generation who were fortunate enough to attend the lectures of that great personality Sir Michael Foster, who habitually emphasised the salient points of his discourse by a rhythmical pronation of his right wrist.

I have said enough to indicate the interest which would attach to a complete analysis of the mental levels which would be obscured or which would remain after exposure to varying degrees of oxygen want.

Alcohol affects different persons in different ways: so on my journeyings in high altitudes I have seen most of the symptoms of alcoholism reproduced. I have seen men vomit, I have seen them quarrel, I have seen them become reckless, I have seen them become garrulous, I have seen them become morose. I have seen one of the most disciplined of men shout and fling his arms about on the edge of a crevasse to the great embarrassment of the guide. I have seen the most loyal companion become ill-tempered and abusive to the point at which I feared international complications. So much for the similarity between acute oxygen want and drunkenness. Let me pass to the comparison between chronic oxygen want and fatigue.

During my stay of six days in the chamber at Cambridge I carried out a number of tests suggested by Mr Bartlett of the Department of Psychology at Cambridge. The research was extended by Dr Lowson who went into the matter much more fully, and lastly we carried out systematic tests in Peru. Any work done so far must be regarded as of a preliminary character. The judgment which I am inclined to pass upon it at present is as follows: the specific mental tests used have shown conspicuously little difference between the qualities of mind at high and low altitudes. Yet I am not prepared to admit that our mental capacity was the same at Cerro as it is here. All the party will agree, I believe, that the reason why the mental tests failed to reveal the difference was because our mental disability was of too subtle a character to be revealed by somewhat simple tests than because the fitness of our minds was unimpaired. It is possible to force oneself to do good work even though the test measures the quality of work done; but were it ideal it would also measure the degree of concentration brought to bear upon the task.

The tests which Mr Doggart practised upon us were as follows:

(1) A memory test. A number consisting of ten integers written on a card was exposed for a given time and then removed from view. The subject was required to write down the number from memory. The test was repeated ten times. There was no certain difference in the correctness of the answers at Cerro and at the sea-level.

(2) A multiplication test which consisted in the doing of a sum such as
$$21786 \times 81345.$$

Speaking for myself, all I can say is that I did the sums about equally badly at different altitudes. Prof. Meakins and Mr Doggart were somewhat less efficient at Cerro, but not very markedly so. And yet experience shows that in daily life one is more stupid over one's arithmetic at high altitudes. I am convinced that could I find the ordinary scribbling paper on which laboratory sums were worked out at Cerro de Pasco, there would be many more mistakes on a sheet than there would be on a similar sheet of working here. There are two explanations for this conviction. The first assumes the conviction to be correct, the second assumes the conviction to be incorrect. If arithmetic as a whole is done as correctly here as at Cerro, my conviction to the contrary may be explained by the supposition that I have transferred the great subjective feeling of difficulty in doing the arithmetic into a belief in the inferior objective quality of the accomplishment. The more likely explanation, I think, is that when one is doing the multiplication test at Cerro one makes the necessary effort of concentration sufficient to do the test with the same degree of accuracy which one can attain elsewhere, but that in the ordinary routine of laboratory arithmetic one does not make any such special effort, with the result that the arithmetic is badly done. Apart from the actual processes of addition, subtraction, etc., there seemed to be an unwonted difficulty in stating a sum at Cerro if it were not of a quite simple character. The Van Slyke method of gas analysis demands the application of some rather complicated tables of correction to the gas volumes as actually measured. These corrections loomed large at Cerro altogether out of proportion to their real difficulty.

I am not sure that a good test would not be some form of algebra— the solution of some problems. If papers in algebra and geometry could be so designed as to take the usual three hours and to be of such a character that the examinee would get about 50–70 per cent. on it under normal circumstances; it would be interesting to confront him with it at Cerro.

The Alphabet Test consisted in placing 27 letters indiscriminately on the table. These included each letter of the alphabet, together with one letter which was reduplicated. The test consisted in measuring the length of time which elapsed before the experimenter discovered which letter was reduplicated. The test, however, yielded no very definite difference—at different altitudes.

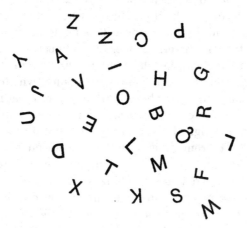

FIG. 51. The alphabet with the letter L reduplicated.

The Clock Test was the one test which with me gave a definite result. The test consisted in being suddenly shown a clock, either of the ordinary type or one so made as to resemble the reversed image of a clock, i.e., what a clock would look like in a mirror. The hands could be put where the tester chose. The time was taken between the exposure of the clock and the receipt of a correct answer.

		Reversed face	Ordinary face	Difference
Sea-level	... ...	5 minutes	2·6 minutes	2·4 minutes
Matucana	... ...	8 ,,	2 ,,	6 ,,
Cerro	... ...	10 ,,	1·6 ,,	8·4 ,,

My reaction to the ordinary clock was faster whilst that to the reversed clock was slower. And this brings me to the similarity between chronic oxygen want and fatigue, for in fatigue there is at first a heightening of mental processes to simple reactions.

Prof. Meakins did not experience the same difficulty at high altitudes in telling the time by the reversed clock—a fact which raises some reflections of interest. The drawback about the test is that after you have done it a few times you get into a system which enables you to elude the process of reversing the clock in your mind. Once this occurs, the particular point which you are trying to test is eliminated.

At Montreal, where Prof. Meakins graduated, there was in the Student's Club a mirror, in the mirror a clock could be seen from a certain position. The students used to indulge in the following pastime. When a group of students suddenly came in sight of the clock one would ask the others the time, the one who first answered correctly was "stood" a drink by his friends. This being so, it appeared that from long practice the reversed clock was almost as easy for him to read as the direct clock, i.e., he read it almost reflexly and never performed in his mind the process of reversing, which was what in my case took the time. On the other hand, I must admit to having had from childhood more than usual difficulty in knowing the difference between my right hand and my left. Even now if I am asked suddenly I have to remember either the position of a wart which was on my right hand as a child or to place myself at table in the dining room of my old home to think which hand was nearest the window. The same mental defect has always been a difficulty to me when sailing. I am rather apt to say west when I mean east and *vice versa*. Orientation of this type seems to involve for me a more complicated mental process than for most persons, and experience has taught me that mistakes in orientation are much more likely to occur when my mind is fatigued than when it is fresh.

Summing up the impressions obtained from the mental tests as a whole, however, they amounted to this: the effect of altitude showed itself rather in the effort of mind needful to do the test than in the accuracy with which it was done.

The same was true of my mental condition during the experiment (to which I have alluded) in which I spent six days in a glass chamber where the concentration of oxygen was regulated; at the commencement it corresponded to an altitude of about 10,000 feet, at the end to 16,000 feet. During these six days innumerable analyses of the chamber air were made with the Haldane apparatus, and to my great surprise only on one occasion did I make an error in technique, such as getting the soda in one of the taps of the apparatus. Even then the error was but a trifling one. It is improbable that I would carry out the same number of analyses under normal circumstances with fewer errors. There was, however, no comparison between the difficulty of carrying out the analyses in the chamber and in ordinary air. In the chamber a high degree of mental concentration was required during every moment of the work and no doubt the success attained was due to the fact that I was entirely undisturbed. In the laboratory of course to any skilled analyst, if his mind is fresh, much of the routine of gas analysis is little more than a reflex. He can carry on a simple conversation about some quite foreign subject much of the time. "If his mind is fresh"—but often when my mind has not been fresh, I have had to do my gas analysis just as in the chamber, to send everybody out of the room, to lock the door and to focus all my faculties upon the work.

It may, of course, be urged that in the chamber, and with more obvious truth at Cerro de Pasco, one really was suffering from fatigue, and that fatigue, not oxygen want, was the cause of one's mental disability. Chronic oxygen want, like mental fatigue, breeds a mental apathy which may amount merely to carelessness, but which, on the other hand, may go so far as to produce complete distortion of the values of things. Matters of vital importance appear trivial and are neglected. Of this I may give two examples.

Dr Longstaff once told me that in his expedition to the Himalayas he made it one of his principal objects to ascertain the height of the various summits by means of observations with the *theodolite*. When he was observing some of the highest he so far lost interest as not to work out and check the results which he obtained while he was on the ground. He arrived at a lower level and found that the observations of one peak showed it to be higher than Everest. As the observations were unchecked, of course they could not be published, and he was left in a state of uncertainty as to whether he had or had not discovered the highest summit in the world. Of course I am not concerned here with any question of whether Longstaff's peak was or was not a few feet higher than Everest. The point with which I am concerned is that at the moment of its discovery he did not care. Here was one of the main objects of his expedition, namely to discover which summit was actually the highest, he obtained all the figures, and yet had not sufficient interest in them at the time to ascertain the relative heights of the peaks, though had his brain been more fully supplied with oxygen he would have been on the tip-toe of excitement. Lastly, he did not realise the vital point, namely that with his figures unchecked any observations of interest which appeared when the calculations were ultimately made would not be sufficiently reliable to convince either himself or the scientific world.

The second example of more or less chronic anoxæmia leading to indifference to the relative importance of things is furnished by the circumstances which led up to the termination of my six days' experiment in the glass chamber. I had intended to be incarcerated for a week, and, needless to say, I had taken the greatest pains to regulate the composition of the air so that on the one hand it was as free as possible from carbonic acid, and on the other the partial pressure of oxygen was gradually diminishing. The machinery for this purpose did not always work smoothly. On the Thursday (the experiment having commenced on a Sunday) things went very badly, but the difficulties were overcome and all was going well and smoothly on the Saturday morning, by which time the oxygen pressure had dropped to a figure which corresponded to about 18,000 feet, from which point it suddenly went up to one which was the equivalent of 15,000 feet. I was in bed with a bad headache—more fortunate than Longstaff, I had at hand someone with a clearer vision than my own. About noon my wife came to see me and on enquiring as to what the oxygen pressure might be I told her that it had been 18,000 feet but that it had just jumped to 15,000 and I added that "after all it made no difference." She seized the psychological point at once, saw that my judgment of what was important had gone and that the whole experiment was in jeopardy. She therefore represented to my colleagues that if it were to end satisfactorily it had better end soon.

The sequel is perhaps worth recording as illustrating a different point, namely that like mental fatigue, chronic oxygen want undermines that self-control which normally prevents one's feelings from manifesting themselves in exaggerated ways. It was not till all the preparations had been made for the operation with which the experiment was to terminate that my colleague who was in charge medically, told me that the end had come. I commenced to cry—and I never quite knew why. Only once do I remember an occurrence of at all a similar nature in my own experience. It was towards the end of the war, the doctor told me that I must give up work and take a complete rest for a fortnight—so far so good. He also suggested something which under ordinary circumstances I should have found very attractive, namely a fortnight in Ireland with my people. For some reason, which at this distance of time I cannot quite recognise, the thought of a journey broke me down completely and the advent of unexpected tears lead to a welcome change in the suggested treatment—namely a rest at home.

Towards the end of our time at Cerro de Pasco, our minds certainly resembled those of worn-out people. The question which arises in this connection is, were these symptoms due to oxygen want, or did we seem worn out simply because of fatigue? It is necessary to enquire whether the same strain would have produced the same effects at the sea-level. It is certain that, with perhaps the exception of myself, all the party worked at Cerro very hard and for long hours. It is certain that they were worked to a standstill, for on the last two or three days of our residence the quality of our work fell very much. I think, but this is only a personal opinion, that a holiday at Cerro would have done little good and that if it had been necessary for us to undertake a further big block of work, we would have had to descend to lower altitudes for a holiday to "pull ourselves together." The symptoms of a tired mind were very obvious to me at the end of my six days in the chamber. I was aphasic, short in the temper and lacking in self-control to a remarkable extent—quite trifling occurrences made me furious. My food used to be put in through a trap-door. I remember being beside myself because my attendant put in the whole paraphernalia for dinner, cruets, changes of silver, etc. (as indeed was her duty), when in my view very much less would have done. Most people with tired minds will understand these unreasoning brain storms. It could not be said that I worked hard in the chamber.

The experience of residents at Cerro de Pasco is definitely that concentrated thought is more fatiguing to the mind there than at the sea-level. It was put to me in this way. Accountancy (which I suppose is largely mechanical) is done up to the same standard at Cerro as in New York, but the drafting of a complicated report at Cerro on which the important financial decisions hinge, involves a degree of mental wear sufficient to demand a holiday "trip to the coast."

The comparison between the effects of altitude and those of fatigue become very difficult at this point because of the sleep factor, or rather the sleeplessness factor. Of course, at first sight the comparison is easy: sleeplessness is a symptom both of mental fatigue and of chronic oxygen want. In the glass case experiment I had the opportunity of judging a little more exactly of anoxæmic sleeplessness than is usually the case. A committee of undergraduate pupils of mine made up their minds that I was never to be left alone, two of them therefore sat up each night outside the case lest help of any sort should be required. I used to ask them in the morning how I had slept, and each morning except perhaps the last they said I had slept well. My own view of the matter was quite otherwise. I thought I had been awake half the night and was unrefreshed in the morning. I was conscious of their moving about and looking in through the glass to see whether or not I was awake. I used to count my pulse at intervals. The two opinions can only be reconciled on the hypothesis that whilst I spent most of the night in sleep, the slumber was very light and fitful with incessant dreams. Even some low degree of consciousness which fell short of absolute wakefulness. At Cerro it was the same: measured in hours we slept well, but the quality of the sleep in most cases was of an inferior order. The night seemed long and we woke unrefreshed.

The reader will now see the difficulty in which we are placed, hard work on the mountain top associated with this type of insomnia is very wearing to the mind, and it is therefore quite open to contention that our mental condition when we left Cerro was really fatigue caused by the combination of activity with the inferior quality of sleep. If so, we would have fallen into a vicious circle in which the fatigue would soon have accentuated the sleeplessness. Here the question may be left.

Before closing I should like to make my position clear about one point. I should like to disabuse the mind of an idea which might perhaps be read into my remarks, namely that mental fatigue is due to oxygen want. There is no real evidence for or against such a view. If the two causes produce the same effect it is not unnatural to suppose that they are connected. Inasmuch, however, as the working of the mind, like that of the body, is ultimately dependent upon the oxidation of specific substances, it is clear that the impairment of the minds actively might be brought about by a defect in any link in the oxidation process—deficiency in quantity or quality of oxidisable material, deficiency in catalyst or deficiency in oxygen. Looked at from this point of view, deficiency of oxygen might produce the same general result as excessive use. From another angle the following statement might be held to sum up the facts. A given strain produces a greater degree of mental fatigue (as it would of muscle fatigue) when the oxygen supply is deficient than when it is ample.

BIBLIOGRAPHY

(1) SCHNEIDER. *Physiological Reviews*, I. 631. 1921.
(2) FOSTER AND HALDANE. *The Investigation of Mine Air*, 177. London, 1905.
(3) HALDANE, KELLAS AND KENNAWAY. *Journ. Physiol.* LIII. 181. 1919.

CHAPTER XIII

ACCLIMATISATION

WITHIN the century or more since scientific men first studied on themselves the effect of ascent into high altitudes, the centre of interest has undergone a great change. Formerly, observation was focussed on the immediate effects of atmospheric rarity, now research is concentrated rather on the mechanism by which the human body becomes acclimatised to its surroundings, so that in the majority of persons, after a short residence at such an altitude as evokes mountain sickness, the more acute symptoms disappear and the more chronic ones become mitigated. The nausea, vomiting, headache, nose-bleeding, hardness of hearing and the dimness of vision, no longer are experienced, and the palpitation and breathlessness become much reduced.

How does such a change take place?

The consideration of acclimatisation must start from the fact that on arrival at high altitudes both the quantity and the pressure of oxygen in the blood which feeds the tissues become deficient. Of these two, the quantity and the pressure, the latter is the important factor, the former matters in so far as it affects the latter. For the ultimate deficiency is a deficiency of oxygen reaching the cell, and the quantity of oxygen which reaches the cell depends, among other things, on the pressure of oxygen in the plasma.

Sooner or later, preferably sooner, the symptoms caused by deficiency of oxygen become less marked. How this takes place is not at all evident. There has been a disposition in physiological thought to suppose that a simple answer can be given to such a question. A philosophy of that type has no attraction for me as being one which bears a close relation to the facts. Far rather would I put forward the hypothesis that when a complex alters, every component in the complex undergoes a change in order to fit in its fellow.

Let us summarise the factors which, so far as our party could discover, contributed to acclimatisation. Of these the first is increased total ventilation due to the effect of oxygen want in the respiratory centre. In discussing this question in Chapter VII I pointed out an intellectual difficulty—that of regarding the lack of anything as an irritant. Oxygen deficiency would dull a fire and *a priori* one might expect it to have a similar effect on the brain. Deficient oxidation may lead to the formation of some toxic substance which heightens the irritability of the centre perhaps before ultimately deadening it. Again respiration may be subject normally to a species of inhibition which is removed. Whatever the mechanism, the fact that a greater quantity of air ventilates the lung at high altitudes than at low ones, seems to be beyond doubt.

In the case of visitors to the mountains this increased ventilation is attained by increasing the respiratory movements. In the case of the Indians one must also consider the increased size of the chest. As will be shown later, the value of heightened ventilation is that it increases the quantity of air passing through the lungs relatively to the quantity of carbonic acid produced. Thus if a man could put an infinitely large volume of air through his lungs per minute, the amount of carbonic acid in the alveoli would be infinitely small, so rapidly would it be swept away, and the amount of oxygen in the same would not differ appreciably from that in the atmosphere breathed except in so far as it was reduced by dilution with aqueous vapour.

In the case of the small bodied but large chested Cholos, one may suppose that the quantities of oxygen used and CO_2 given out are proportional in quantity to the body surface (as compared with similar measurements in the white races), but that the ventilation of the lungs is at least as great as that of an Anglo-Saxon of five feet and ten inches tall. If this were so, it would follow that the alveolar air of the Cholo had a low CO_2 content, and just in proportion as the CO_2 was low the oxygen approximated to that of the atmosphere.

To return to the Anglo-Saxon, the effect of increased ventilation as a factor in acclimatisation is well shown by a comparison of the alveolar airs of Douglas and myself in Teneriffe[1]. Douglas thus gained the advantage over me of about 10 mm., an amount which at the top of the Peak was about 20 per cent. of the whole oxygen tension in the alveolar air. That was no small advantage.

Such an alteration cannot take place without the appearance of consequential changes in other systems, for the fall in the pressure of carbonic acid in the alveolar air is reflected in the blood where there is a corresponding drop in CO_2 content. Such a drop, if no other change took place, would raise the alkalinity of the blood and presumably would tend to decrease the ventilation and abolish the degree of acclimatisation which takes place. It may therefore be supposed that at high altitudes, as Haldane, Kellas and Kennaway[2] have shown to be the case under artificial conditions, the kidney secreted bicarbonate and it is certain that a considerable percentage of the bicarbonate present disappears from the blood. So much for the changes which can be referred directly to the effect of oxygen want upon the respiratory centre.

Another factor in acclimatisation which appears to be consequent upon the diminished oxygen in the arterial blood is the rise in the quantity of hæmoglobin in each cubic centimetre of blood, and eventually in the body as a whole. The mechanism of this change is quite obscure. The question may first be raised: Is the alteration due to diminution of oxygen pressure or of oxygen content in the arterial blood? To this question the Pike's Peak Expedition (1911)(3) gives an unequivocal answer that the cause is diminished oxygen pressure. The reason given is the very cogent one, the increase of hæmoglobin may be so great as to cause an actual increase in the oxygen content of the blood even though there is a fall in the percentage of oxygen as compared with total hæmoglobin. Yet it must not be forgotten that if the oxygen content of the arterial blood is reduced without reducing the pressure, as may be done by the administration of carbon monoxide, an exactly similar increase in the hæmoglobin value of the blood is described. In both cases there is a fall in the average concentration of oxygen in the plasma of the capillaries and this is probably the important point.

Whether the concentration of corpuscles in the blood is caused by abstraction of water or by an absolute increase in the number of red cells has been frequently discussed. Here there is no real antithesis because the two processes are not mutually exclusive. It was shown quite clearly by Douglas, Haldane, Henderson and Schneider that the total amount of hæmoglobin in the body increased on Pike's Peak and that, roughly speaking, the increase in the hæmoglobin value of the blood was due to the introduction of fresh hæmoglobin into the circulation. Whether at the commencement of residence at high altitude there is a fall in the blood volume is less certain. The hypothesis that the first stage in the increase in the "blood count" is heralded in by an absorption of water is fascinating, but at present it is ill-supported by evidence. Data which support it appeared in one of the four cases studied on Pike's Peak (3). Even in that case the blood volume, shortly after arrival at the summit, was little below what it had been normally at Oxford. There seems also to be a temperature factor in the measurement of the blood volume which it is difficult to separate from the altitude factor. The dilemma in which we are placed is this: granted that hæmoglobin is not formed as rapidly as it makes its appearance in the blood, and that there is little evidence of concentration by the abstraction of water from the plasma, whence can the hæmoglobin come? Is there any store in the body which can contribute a little to assist in tiding matters over until the supply is put on a proper footing by increased manufacture. One such store seems to exist and it may not be the only one. Recent work in the Cambridge laboratory seems to indicate (1) that normally most of the hæmoglobin in the spleen is outside the circulation (4), (2) that anoxæmic conditions cause a contraction of the spleen which may amount to half of its own volume. It seems possible that the spleen may, in this way, add 100 cubic centimetres of corpuscles to the circulation or about 5 per cent. of the whole number in circulation. The mechanism of the splenic output is clear, the anoxæmia acts on the central nervous system and causes a stimulation of the spleen through the sympathetic system (5).

Undoubtedly the principal factor in the maintenance of a high hæmoglobin value in the blood is the increased production of cells in the bone marrow. The evidence seems to show that the rate of production increases at least in proportion to the quantity of hæmoglobin present in the body. The figures presented in the Pike's Peak (3) report suggest that the whole increase in the blood volume is accounted for by the addition of corpuscles to the circulation. The average increase of blood volume is 13 per cent., the average increase of hæmoglobin is 32 per cent., granting that the corpuscles constituted initially about 40 per cent. of the whole blood—then 32 per cent. of 40 is 13.

The evidence of new corpuscular formation is to be found not only in an increase in the total hæmoglobin, great beyond anything which could be contributed from the storehouses in the body, but also in the advent of large numbers of reticulated cells to the circulation. These are probably young cells.

Whilst it is easy to observe the excessive quantity of hæmoglobin which makes its appearance in the blood of Europeans who go up into the Andes, and which is normal in the blood of all natives of the really high parts of the world, it is less easy to see the precise use of so large a quantity of pigment. Formerly, the explanation was given that all this hæmoglobin was of use "because it carried more oxygen to the tissues." This in the last resort is probably true, but the difficulty is to see just how the carriage of more oxygen to the tissues is of advantage to them. Already each tissue has on the average three times as much oxygen carried to it as it requires. If, at high altitudes, owing to a 10 per cent. deficiency in the arterial blood, this "3" were reduced to "2·7," that is still a quantity of oxygen far beyond the tissue's needs. It is not deficiency of actual quantity of oxygen in the blood which is the cause of the trouble in the mountains, it is deficiency of the pressure at which the oxygen is transported. The point which needs elucidation is this. How does an increase in the quantity of hæmoglobin in the blood lead to an increase in the average oxygen pressure in the capillary? The answer must be given in two stages and can best be understood if illustrated by a numerical example.

Suppose at the sea-level, the arterial blood which reaches a tissue has an oxygen capacity of ·185 c.c. of oxygen per cubic centimetre of blood, that it is 96 per cent. saturated and that the tissue takes out 38 per cent. of the oxygen or ·07 c.c. per cubic centimetre of blood. The venous blood is then 58 per cent. saturated and consequently, on the capillary dissociation curve of Christiansen, Douglas and Haldane given below, would have an oxygen pressure of 37 mm. Now let us go up to 14,000 feet, where the arterial blood with normal respiration would be perhaps 83 per cent. saturated and where on the same curve its oxygen will be at a pressure of 53 mm. Assume that still ·07 c.c. of oxygen is taken out of each cubic centimetre of blood and that the reduction in percentage saturation is therefore 38 per cent. as before, the venous blood will be 45 per cent. saturated and its oxygen pressure will be 31 mm. The subject resides at 14,000 feet, and we will suppose that in time his hæmoglobin value rises to 150 instead of 100, so that the oxygen capacity of his blood becomes $·185 \times \frac{150}{100} = ·278$ c.c. Let us go through our calculation again. His arterial blood is 83 per cent. saturated, ·07 c.c. is taken out. Now ·07 is only 25 per cent. of ·278 and therefore the percentage saturation of the venous blood will be $83 - 25 = 58$. This will correspond to a pressure of 37 mm. Tabulating the above partial pressures of oxygen, we have:

	Oxygen pressure in mm.	
	Arterial blood	Venous blood
(1) Sea-level Hb = 100	110	37
(2) Reduced oxygen pressure Hb = 100 ...	53	31
(3) Reduced oxygen pressure Hb = 150 ...	53	37

Now it is clear that taking cases (2) and (3) above, both of which assume the same arterial oxygen pressure, the one which has the higher venous pressure will also have the highest average pressure of oxygen in the capillary. This would be so even if the average capillary pressure were the arithmetic mean of the arterial and venous pressures; all this has been pointed out by other authors, as will be found in the Pike's Peak report(3). What has not been sufficiently stressed is that, as appears usually to be the case, the average pressure in the capillary approximates rather closely to the pressure of oxygen in the vein. An example is worked out in the *Report of the Cerro Expedition*, p. 433[1], in which it is assumed that the pressure in the tissue is but one millimetre below that in the venous blood, that the arterial blood is of the order of 50 or 60 mm. above the average of the tissues, whilst the average pressure in the capillary is about 1·4 mm. above that in the tissues and therefore only ·4 mm. above that in the venous blood. If, on the other hand, there is a difference of pressure of 10 mm. between the oxygen pressure in the tissue and that in the venous blood, there would be something like 13 mm. between the average oxygen pressure in the capillary and that in the tissue, the oxygen pressure in the capillary would therefore average 3 mm. higher than that in the vein, while it would be something like 50 mm. lower than that in the artery. The difficulty in the calculation is that we do not know how nearly the pressure in the tissue approximates to that in the vein. It seems reasonable, however, to say that the average oxygen pressure in the capillary differs only by a few millimetres from that in the vein, hence the importance of any change which raises the venous pressure, such a change as the increase in the hæmoglobin value of the blood. Therefore it comes to pass that, reverting to the three cases tabulated above, the average oxygen pressure in the capillary in case (3) is probably closer to that in case (1) than it is to that in case (2).

Taken separately, we have seen that increased ventilation raises the oxygen pressure in the alveolar air and consequently in the arterial blood, and that increased concentration of hæmoglobin produces a rise of oxygen pressure in the venous blood—but there is a subtler element in acclimatisation which appears to depend upon a combination of the dissipation of carbonic acid from the blood and the concentration of corpuscles. Let me first describe it and then say why

---

[1] See also the work of L. J. Henderson, A. V. Bock, H. Field, Jr. and J. L. Stoddard. *Journ. of Biol. Chem.* LIX. 379.

I attribute it to the causes indicated. That change is the alteration in the dissociation curve, described in Chapter VII, by which the blood gains in its affinity for oxygen and by which therefore it can take up a greater quantity of oxygen at any given pressure short of that necessary for complete saturation.

In our discussion of the dissociation curve we drew attention to the quantity of oxygen which the arterial blood gained at any given pressure. We are here faced with the question, Does the change in the position of the curve affect the pressure of oxygen as well as the quantity? At first sight it might appear that the pressure in the arterial blood is regulated by that in the alveolar air and that in the presence of alveolar air of a certain composition a mere change in the form of the dissociation curve could not alter the pressure of oxygen in the blood. There are possibilities, however, which must not be overlooked. The oxygen pressure in the arterial blood and in the alveolar air are never, on any theory of diffusion, the same. The pressure in the air is the limiting pressure to that in the blood but always exceeds it[1]—possibly by ever so little, a fraction of a milli-metre perhaps, but still in theory there is a margin. We are thrown back to a consideration of the factors which regulate the margin. The principles which underlie these factors are: (1) that taking the whole length of the capillary in the lung, a certain average difference of pressure has to be maintained between the pressure of oxygen in the air and that in the capillary, and (2) the greater the quantity of oxygen absorbed per minute the greater must be the average dif-ference of pressure. Now under normal circumstances, with a pressure of 100 mm. in the lung, and with the venous blood, shall we say again 58 per cent. saturated, it will be clear that the venous blood arrives at the lung with an oxygen pressure very far below that in the alveolus. In the case shown in Fig. 21 a the difference would be $100 - 36 = 64$ mm., and not only so but, owing to the shape of the oxygen dissociation curve, the difference is maintained (not in so great a degree but still to a very large extent) nearly up to the point at which the blood becomes arterial. Thus with a pressure of 60 mm. of mercury, more or less, the oxygen is rapidly driven into the alveolar capillary, in the very first portion of which it becomes almost arterial.

---

[1] I would crave the forgiveness of the school of workers who think otherwise, if I do not argue the point here. It is certainly out of no disrespect for their work, still less for themselves. The reasons on which the above statement is based will be given at length in a companion volume to this on the Theory of Respiration, and it seems redundant to repeat them.

As it traverses the remainder of the capillary it picks up the last traces of oxygen and emerges almost in equilibrium with the alveolar air. Imagine now that the pressure in alveolar air had been but 50 mm. instead of 100 mm. The venous blood would have differed from the alveolar air by only 14 mm. The pressure driving the oxygen into the blood would have been less than the quarter of its previous value, and even this would have dwindled away proportionately at a much greater rate than in the case in which the lung contained normal alveolar air. Thus when the blood reaches the terminal portion of the capillary and disappears into the pulmonary veins it will be less nearly in equilibrium with the alveolar air than is normally the case. Indeed the difference may even become measurable. And if at rest the blood which passes through the lung fails of equilibrium with the alveolar air by a measurable amount the failure will be accentuated in proportion as exercise is taken. These things were found to be so in tests made on Meakins at Cerro de Pasco. One can put the matter in another way, and say that at high altitudes the blood is too short a time in the capillary to reach approximate equilibrium with the alveolar air, or if you will you can say that the capillary is too short for the purpose. The result is that the arterial blood goes to the tissue with an oxygen pressure even lower than the limiting one of the alveolar air, and this deficiency must tell all along the capillary; if the utilisation is unaltered, the blood will emerge from the tissue correspondingly more venous, and the average capillary pressure in the tissue will be correspondingly reduced. Now to revert to the alteration of the dissociation curve, the question we have to answer is: Does this alteration enable the blood, as it passes through the lung, to attain more nearly to the limiting alveolar pressure of oxygen? If the movement of the curve tends to increase the difference in pressure between the oxygen in the blood, at any particular degree of saturation, and that in the alveolar air its effect will be to promote the more rapid diffusion of gas into the blood and the ultimate attainment by the blood of a closer approximation to equilibrium with the air in the alveolus.

This indeed is the effect produced, for as the dissociation curve moves closer to the ordinate (that in sense indicating a lower pressure for any percentage saturation) it follows that at any particular oxygen content the pressure in the blood is further removed from that in the alveolar air. Thus the average difference between the pressures in the air contained in the lung and in the blood which arrives will, other things being equal, be increased. It follows that oxygen passes more rapidly into the blood of the acclimatised than of the unac-climatised person and therefore the blood of the acclimatised individual can more nearly reach an equilibrium with the air of the lung.

In short, the blood of a person whose dissociation curve has so shifted, will, after traversing the lung capillary, start on its journey to the tissue laden with a greater amount of oxygen at a higher pressure than was the case with the unshifted curve.

There is however another side to the benefits which the body can derive from the acquisition of a greater affinity for oxygen by the blood. True, the hæmoglobin picks up the oxygen more rapidly in the lung, but just in proportion as it does so it parts with the oxygen less rapidly in the tissues and it may be argued that as the goal and end of oxygen transport is the feeding of the tissues, the body so far from being at an advantage is at a disadvantage. This argument has much in it which will repay consideration, but let us point out that the oxygen cannot get out of the blood unless it first gets into it. Then let us concede that the tissues are at a disadvantage, all that can be contended is that they are at a less disadvantage under the new circumstances where the oxygen is more readily acquired by the blood and imparted less readily than they would be if the blood acquired the oxygen in less quantity and under less pressure, even though it could impart it more easily.

And this redistribution of disadvantages appears to be the real essence of acclimatisation. The acclimatised man is not the man who has attained to bodily and mental powers as great in Cerro de Pasco as he would have in Cambridge (whether that town be situated in Massachussetts or in England). Such a man does not exist. All dwellers at high altitudes are persons of impaired physical and mental powers. The acclimatised man is he who is least impaired, or, in other words, he who has made least demand upon his reserve. At rest he will appear like the dweller on the plain, but exercise will always bring him to a standstill sooner at the higher altitude.

The most completely acclimatised man is he whose system can distribute the extra strain most evenly over the whole organism so that no one part will give way before any other.

The readjustment of the load between the blood and the tissues is shown by the movement of the dissociation curve, but it is only an incident in the whole phenomenon of acclimatisation, for, as has been indicated, the whole process is one which ramifies over the entire range of the body's functions. If one sits down to answer the question whether or not anything remains absolutely unaltered at high altitudes, it is not an easy matter to find one such function. The respiration alters, which is a way of saying that the degree of muscular contraction alters; as the constitution of the urine alters, the work of the kidney presumably alters also; the pulse alters, which throws a strain on the heart and this strain may be met to some extent by variations in the vascular system: but there is one possible alteration which has not been taken into account by any party of workers on high altitude and that is the blood supply to the brain.

The modes of acclimatisation which we have discussed have been for the most part such as affect the body as a whole. Yet it must not be forgotten that the burden of the symptoms which together are called mountain sickness are not symptoms of the body as a whole but symptoms of the brain. The more acute are symptoms of one portion of the brain, a mass of tissue perhaps the size of a pea, which is situated in the medulla oblongata and which contains the "centres" for cardiac inhibition, vomiting, vaso-motor tone and the like. Surely if we are on the look-out for some special mechanism for acclimatisation here is the place in which to search, and the most acute symptoms of mountain sickness are due to oxygen want in the medulla. Such being the case, I have wondered recently that more attention has not been drawn to the fact, and that stress has not been laid on the most simple mechanism for increasing the oxygen supply to that important locality. Such, surely, would be an increase in its blood supply.

It may be that the once prevalent doctrine of the absence of vaso-motor fibres to the brain diverted men's minds from the possibility of medullary hyperæmia as a factor in acclimatisation, but as I once heard Prof. Langley point out, the evidence for this doctrine in no way precludes a vaso-motor supply to the medulla. Moreover, the recent work of Roberts [6] which has matured since our return from Peru, has supplied much positive evidence that, whatever may be said of the higher parts of the brain, the medulla, at all events, has a vaso-motor supply. It may be that before the work of Krogh men's minds were less alive to the extent to which alterations of the blood supply and especially the opening up of fresh vessels, could increase the oxygen pressure in a tissue. But whatever the reason, the fact remains that any explanation of acclimatisation which leaves the blood supply of the medulla out of account, falls short at the precise point at which the maximum of acclimatisation might be sought with the probable minimum of dislocation of function. Yet even if the medulla were relieved by an increased local supply of oxygen, it would only be to bring oxygen want nearer to the tissues as a whole, to broaden as it were the basis of taxation on the body.

It is no part of my philosophy to suppose that this or that function of the body is kept constant by a process of sweating its fellows, and as far as I can see such a doctrine is quite unsupported by facts. The oxygen in the arterial blood does not remain constant, the CO_2 pressure in the alveolar air does not remain constant, the hydrogen-ion concentration of the blood does not remain constant—but they and a score of other things settle down to form a new equilibrium. If artificially one is altered the rest alter in unison. If I may be allowed a rough analogy, it is as though a new tax were imposed; say an addition to the income tax. It appears to be paid by a group of persons with large incomes, in reality, by reason of alteration in prices, unemployment and the like, it is spread over the whole population, and the more completely and justly it is spread the less the strain on the community.

This is no new doctrine—it has been stated in words that have come through the ages: "If one member suffer all the members suffer with it....the whole body fitly joined together and compacted by that which every joint supplieth according to the effectual working in the measure of every part maketh increase of the body to the edifying of itself."

BIBLIOGRAPHY

(1) BARCROFT. *Journ. Physiol.* XLII. 44. 1911.

(2) HALDANE, KELLAS AND KENNAWAY. *Journ. Physiol.* LIII. 180. 1919.

(3) DOUGLAS, HALDANE, HENDERSON AND SCHNEIDER. *Phil. Trans. Roy. Soc.* B. CCIII. 185. 1913.

(4) BARCROFT, J. AND H. *Journ. Physiol.* LVIII. 138. 1923. Also HANAK AND HARKAVY. *Journ. Physiol.* LIX. 121. 1924. And BARCROFT, J. *The Lancet.* 14 Feb, 1925. p. 319.

(5) DE BOER AND CARROLL. *Journ. Physiol.* LIX. 312. 1924.

(6) ROBERTS, Ff. *Journ. Physiol.* LV. 346. 1921; and LVII. 405. 1922.

APPENDIX I

PHYSIOLOGICAL DIFFICULTIES IN THE ASCENT OF MOUNT EVEREST

MAJOR R. W. G. HINGSTON, I.M.S.

Medical Officer to the Expedition of 1924

(Reprinted from *The Geographical Journal*, vol. LXV, pp. 4–16)

THE primary object of the Mount Everest Expedition was to reach the highest summit on the Earth. Everything else was subordinate to this. Elaborate scientific investigations were impossible, and anything involving complicated apparatus was altogether out of the question. We had to content ourselves with simple experiments and with the records of the experiences of individual climbers. These, nevertheless, may be worth discussion. They will give us some idea of the physiological difficulties involved in an ascent to so great a height.

ALTERATIONS IN BREATHING

The most obvious of these is the difficulty in breathing. Owing to the gradual nature of our ascent this shortness of respiration was scarcely noticeable below 10,000 feet. It was definitely apparent above 14,000 feet, and above 19,000 feet the slightest exertion made breathing laboured and severe. When the body was at rest, even at extreme altitudes, the rate of breathing was apparently normal and as comfortable as at sea-level. But the very slightest exertion, such as the tying of a bootlace, the opening of a ration-box, the getting into a sleeping-bag, was associated with marked respiratory distress. The difficulties of the ascent were thus enormously increased. The breathing was quicker rather than deeper, but it was necessary to stop at frequent intervals and take a series of long deep breaths. This very quickly brought relief and made one ready for a further advance. Norton told me that, when he found himself dropping behind, his only chance of catching up the party was by taking a number of these deep long breaths. Somervell gives a record of his breathing at 27,000 feet. At that altitude he had to take seven, eight, or ten complete respirations for every single step forward. And even at that slow rate of progress he had to rest for a minute or two every 20 or 30 yards. At 28,000 feet Norton, in an hour's climb, ascended only about 80 feet. This was the highest point reached without the aid of oxygen. The strain at that altitude was certainly intense, but when we remember that the supply of oxygen is only about one-third of that available at sea-level, we are surprised that men can make these strenuous efforts, and still more that they can remain in comparative comfort when they sit down to rest.

The alteration in the rhythm of the breathing—commonly known as Cheyne-Stokes respiration—was frequently noticed during the expedition. I heard one member of the party breathing in this way as low as 12,000 feet. Though as a rule it seldom occurs when awake, yet at the base camp I was conscious of this type of breathing before passing off to sleep. Illness at high altitudes markedly increases it. It was most pronounced in one member when suffering from fever at 15,000 feet, and still more so in a Gurkha when dying of cerebral haemorrhage at 18,000 feet. The rapid breathing of cold dry air produces some important secondary effects. It causes inflammation of the respiratory passages. Every member suffered from sore throat, from hoarseness, or from loss of voice. Most had irritating coughs, but with little expectoration. Some of the porters developed severe bronchitis: one had a profusely ulcerated throat, another persistently coughed up blood. Dr Kellas was of opinion that the breathing was less laboured in a high wind. He thought that the wind might have the effect of packing the air into the lungs; also that it swept away the exhaled air and thus prevented it from being inhaled by the next breath. Our experiences did not agree with his. Mount Everest is noted for its heavy winds. They caused considerable obstruction to the breathing. A moderate breeze had a freshening effect, but a strong wind impeded progress, and there was a feeling of suffocation when facing powerful gusts.

I made some experiments on the respiration. The power of holding the breath is a simple test to which pilots are submitted in the Royal Air Force. The following table shows the diminution in this power at successive altitudes in the ascent. The first column is the most complete. Where at sea-level the breath was held for 64 seconds, at 21,000 feet it was held for only 14 seconds.

Altitude in feet	Time breath held (in secs.)									
	R.W.H.	E.O.S.	B.B.	G.B.	E.F.N.	G.L.M.	J.V.H.	A.C.I.	T.H.S.	N.E.O.
Sea-level	64	—	120	—	—	—	90	120	—	—
7000	40	40	60	40	40	50	42	80	60	55
14,300	39 ·	32	35	32	37	40	90	47	48	—
16,500	20	23	35	20	31	—	23	30	41	28
21,000	14	17	—	20	—	—	17	—	—	—

Another test used amongst airmen is the measurement of the expiratory force. This consists in blowing a column of mercury up a graduated glass tube. The height reached by the mercury is read off, and this gives a measure of the expiratory force. If the expiratory force is much below the average it suggests that the airman will be incapable of sustained effort. The following table gives the results of our experiments. It suggests that with increasing altitude the expiratory force tends to improve. Look again at the first column. At sea-level the expiratory force was 110 mm. Hg; at 21,000 feet it was 150 mm. Hg. The third, fourth, fifth, sixth, seventh and eighth columns also show that an improvement has occurred.

Altitude in feet	Expiratory force in mm. of Hg.									
	R.W.H.	E.O.S.	B.B.	G.B.	E.F.N.	G.L.M.	J.V.H.	A.C.I.	T.H.S.	N.E.O.
Sea-level	110	—	—	—	—	—	—	—	—	—
7000	110	120	140	160	110	110	130	160	120	110
14,300	110	90	160	190	120	120	—	160	120	—
16,500	140	130	210	200	170	—	120	170	120	100
21,000	150	120	—	210	—	—	150	—	—	—

I did not anticipate this improvement in the expiratory force. But the test has little to do with the function of respiration. It is more an indication of physical fitness and muscular strength. And this tends to improve during an ascent, when the progress is slow enough to be accompanied with acclimatisation and before the wasting of high altitudes becomes marked. The march across Tibet made us tougher and harder. Hence the expiratory force improved. Mosso came to a similar conclusion in the Alps. He made his men perform exercises with dumb-bells, and was surprised to find that they did much more work at a height of 4560 metres than when they performed the same exercises at Turin.

CIRCULATION

I pass to the changes in the circulation. Blueness of the face and lips, lividity of the nails, coldness of the extremities, were the indications noticed of the impaired circulation at altitudes above 19,000 feet. Three of the members experienced giddiness. One noticed that it was immediately relieved by taking a deep breath. Once the extremities become cold at these high altitudes there is a great difficulty in regaining warmth even in the interior of a sleeping-bag. The pulse is not markedly accelerated while at rest, but increases rapidly on the slightest exertion. Norton's normal pulse is 40, and it was only 60 when he was resting at 27,600 feet. An intermittent pulse may develop at high altitudes. In one instance, after crossing a pass of only 14,000 feet the pulse missed four beats every minute without causing any particular symptoms of distress. This irregularity of the pulse seems to be a common feature. Mosso states that, when on Monte Rosa, he noticed that nearly all the members of his party showed some signs of irregularity of the heart. Haemorrhages at high altitudes have often been described, from the gums, the lips, the conjunctivae, the nose. Nothing of the kind occurred amongst the members of our expedition.

The following table shows the changes in the pulse of one individual at successive altitudes above sea-level. The first column gives the pulse-rate when the person is at rest. There is no change except at the highest altitude, 21,000 feet. The second column shows the change that occurs when the person is made to stand up. There is an increase in the pulse-rate somewhat in proportion to the altitude of the experiment. Column 3 shows the change after regulated exercise. The exercise consisted in standing alternately on a chair and on the ground five times in 15 seconds.

Again there is a marked increase in the pulse-rate, and this increase is greater the greater the altitude. The last column gives the time in seconds that the pulse takes to return to normal.

Pulse-rate of one individual

Altitude in feet	Pulse-rate per minute sitting	Pulse-rate per minute standing	Pulse-rate per minute after regulated exercise	Time in secs. of return of pulse to normal
Sea-level	72	72	84	20
7000	72	84	96	15
14,300	72	84	108	40
16,500	72	96	120	20
21,000	108	120	144	20

The blood pressure was taken with a sphygmomanometer in the manner adopted by the Royal Air Force. The following is a table of results. There seems to be no change in the blood pressure definitely associated with increase in height.

Blood pressure at successive altitudes

Altitude in feet	R.W.H. Sys.	R.W.H. Dias.	E.O.S. Sys.	E.O.S. Dias.	B.B. Sys.	B.B. Dias.	G.P. Sys.	G.P. Dias.	E.F.N. Sys.	E.F.N. Dias.	J.V.H. Sys.	J.V.H. Dias.	G.L.M. Sys.	G.L.M. Dias.	A.C.I. Sys.	A.C.I. Dias.	T.H.S. Sys.	T.H.S. Dias.	N.E.O. Sys.	N.E.O. Dias.
Sea-level	120	80	—	—	—	—	—	—	—	—	—	—	—	—	—	—	—	—	—	—
7000	130	90	125	90	150	110	130	90	140	80	120	100	120	85	130	100	119	85	100	80
14,300	135	95	115	80	145	85	130	90	135	90	—	—	120	90	130	100	130	90	—	—
16,500	146	104	128	90	140	102	128	93	136	96	126	94	122	78	140	110	120	82	125	95
21,000	138	118	100	80	—	—	110	90	—	—	100	80	—	—	—	—	—	—	—	—

A well-known change that takes place during an ascent to high altitudes is the increase in the number of red corpuscles per unit volume of blood. The conditions on Everest were too rough for these delicate determinations. But further west, on the Pamir plateau, I had previously made a series of blood counts up to 18,203 feet. The following table shows the results:

Date	Altitude (feet)	Corpuscles per cu. mm.
April 10	700	4,480,000
May 12	4,390	5,240,000
May 21	8,000	6,040,000
May 28	10,000	6,624,000
May 30	11,960	6,760,000
June 1	12,400	6,800,000
June 21	13,300	7,525,000
June 23	15,600	7,840,000
June 26	16,900	7,640,000
July 27	18,200	8,320,000

There has been an increase in the number of red corpuscles from 4,480,000 at 700 feet to 8,320,000 at 18,200 feet. Another point of interest is that the people who live on the Central Asian plateau have a higher blood count than those at sea-level. The average blood count of the Sarikoli is 7,596,000, of the Kirghiz 7,920,000. The blood count of the European is about 5,000,000, but, on making an ascent to the Tibetan plateau, the corpuscles in his blood rapidly increase until they reach the number normal to the people who live permanently at those heights.

MUSCULAR POWER

Airmen describe great muscular weakness when flying at considerable altitudes. Even working a camera-shutter calls for enormous effort. We did not notice such pronounced effects, probably because our ascent was slow. But if inhalation is inadequate the legs soon become tired. It is not the tiredness of a prolonged walk, but more a heaviness and a lassitude which quickly disappears with a short rest.

The endurance test employed by the Royal Air Force is said to indicate the stability of the medullary centres and the capacity of the individual to resist fatigue. The test consists in blowing a column of mercury to a height of 40 mm. and noting how long the person is able to sustain it at that height. The pulse is counted in periods of five seconds during the performance of the test. The following table gives the results of this test. Every column shows a diminution in the powers of endurance at each successive height. Take, for example, the first column. At sea-level the subject could sustain the mercury for 45 seconds; at 21,000 feet for only 15 seconds.

Endurance test

Altitude in feet	Time in secs. Hg maintained at 40 mm.									
	R.W.H.	E.O.S.	B.B.	G.B.	E.F.N.	G.L.M.	J.V.H.	A.C.I.	T.H.S.	N.E.O.
Sea-level	45	—	—	—	—	—	—	—	—	—
7000	35	30	60	50	20	60	35	45	50	50
14,300	30	30	25	40	25	35	—	45	25	—
16,500	23	23	23	15	23	—	17	25	22	20
21,000	15	15	—	15	—	—	10	—	—	—

The pulse-rate was taken during the above test. Some of the results are given below. The first figure in each series shows the normal rate of the pulse during the five seconds before the test begins. This figure is separated from the following figures by a stroke. The following figures give the pulse-rate during each successive period of five seconds throughout the performance of the test. Take, for example, the first line of figures in the first column—6/7.8.9.9.8.7. The 6 is the pulse-rate during the five seconds immediately before the test. The 7 is the pulse-rate during the first five seconds of the test. The remaining figures, 8.9.9.8.7, are the pulse-rates during the successive periods of five seconds until the test ends. In this way we obtain the character of the pulse while the person is undergoing continuous strain.

Pulse-rate in seconds during Endurance test

Altitude in feet	E.O.S.	B.B.	G.B.	A.C.I.
7000	6/7.8.9.9.8.7	6/6.7.9.9.9.7.6.6.6.5	5/6.6.8.6.5.4.5.5.5	8/9.11.10.8.7.6.6.6.6
14,300	6/6.7.7.7.7.7	6/7.8.8.6.5	5/7.7.7.6.8.6.5.5	8/9.9.11.10.9.9.9.9.8
16,500	6/7.7.8.7	6/9.9.9.3	6/7.8.9	8/11.10.9.7.6
21,000	8/10.8.6	—	9/10.10.6	—

The chief points of interest in this experiment is the marked slowing of the pulse that takes place when the capacity of endurance is beginning to tell. At the commencement of the test the pulse first increases, but after a lapse of 15 to 20 seconds it begins definitely to slow up. This slowing of the pulse is more marked at the higher altitudes. There is an extreme case in the lowest line of figures of column 2. The 6/9.9.9.3 indicates that on the commencement of the experiment the pulse immediately rushed up from 6 to 9 beats in the first five seconds, and after a lapse of 15 seconds suddenly fell back from 9 to 3. This occurred at 16,500 feet.

Nevertheless, in spite of these vagaries of the pulse, it is remarkable how well the strength is maintained at altitudes over 20,000 feet. This specially strikes us when we observe how animals can move so freely at such great heights. Ravens and crows used to come to our camp at 21,000 feet. We saw lammergeyers circling round the mountain at 23,000 feet, and choughs followed the climbers to their highest bivouac at 27,000 feet. They moved through the air with perfect ease, though it must have required much greater effort to sustain them than when flying in the denser atmosphere of the plains.

SPECIAL SENSES

Changes in the function of the special senses have occasionally been noticed by mountaineers. They describe an impairment of vision, a diminution in hearing, alterations in the taste and smell. Most of our party noticed nothing in this respect, but two members were particularly emphatic in their loss of the sense of taste. One said that "taste was distinctly affected," that "things seemed to have less taste, though there was no change in the character of the flavour." He was unable to taste onions at 19,000 feet. Another found food "distinctly tasteless." At 19,000 feet he could eat a slab of peppermint without strongly appreciating the flavour. Their sense of taste returned on descending to the base camp at 16,500 feet.

PAIN

The only kind of pain which we could attribute to high altitude was the occasional occurrence of a slight headache. Most of the members never experienced it, but some of us noticed it on first reaching the plateau, though, after a few days' acclimatisation, it completely disappeared. It usually commenced at the back of the neck, spread into a general mild headache, and disappeared after an hour's rest. Exercise, and particularly stooping, increased it. Lying down quickly brought relief. Our porters also suffered from headache. Many of them asked for headache tablets the first time we passed over into Tibet. Even the inhabitants of the plateau are not immune. It is common to see patches of plaster on their temples and black pigment smeared on their cheeks. These are remedies which they use to alleviate the headache caused by the altitude and wind.

Gastro-intestinal Symptoms

Loss of appetite is a serious consequence of residence at great heights. Probably it is the cause of much of the wasting that occurs. There is much individual variation in this respect. Some of the climbers maintained that there was no loss of appetite. I found some dislike for food even at the base camp, though this disappeared on acclimatisation. Bruce thought that his appetite was unimpaired up to 21,000 feet. At 23,000 feet he found a disinclination for meat, though he still had an appetite for cereals and sweets. At 25,000 feet he lost all appetite for solid food, but could still take coffee and to a less degree soup. Somervell at 27,000 feet found an absolute distaste for solids, though he enjoyed liquids and sweets and fruit. The general opinion seemed to be that sweet things were the most palatable and meat the least palatable about 19,000 feet. There was no suggestion of nausea or vomiting even at the highest altitudes reached.

Diarrhoea is not uncommon. It is usually of a transient nature, and may be associated with much bile. Occasionally it may be more persistent, and refuse to yield to any treatment until a descent is made to moderate heights. Thirst is a far more important factor. It may be excessive at the end of a hard day, and, owing to the practical difficulties in obtaining water, may cause exhaustion of the climbers and failure of the climb. How best to relieve thirst at the high camps is a most important practical point. The craving for drink is not the result of perspiration, but of the loss of moisture in the respiratory passages from the excessive inhalation of cold dry air. This desiccation of the body at extreme altitudes may result in a great scantiness of urine. One of the climbers at 21,000 feet did not micturate for 16 to 18 hours; another on his descent from 28,000 feet did not do so for 24 hours.

Mental Effects

High altitudes affect the operations of the mind. One member was confident of a dulling of the will power, a diminution in the strength of purpose, with less and less desire to reach the summit the further he made the ascent. Somervell describes a lack of observance at and above 25,000 feet. Bruce records an enfeeblement of memory. He found an effort in recalling previous events. Above 23,000 feet his ideas became increasingly inaccurate. It was necessary for him to record them immediately, as otherwise they would become forgotten or distorted. I think every one experienced some mental lassitude. Though the mind was clear, yet there was a disinclination for effort. It was far more pleasant to sit about than to do a job of work that required thought. We did not notice any peevishness or petulance, though I suspect that high altitudes would cause unsociability in a party less perfectly harmonious than ours. Though mental work is a burden at high altitudes, yet with an effort it can be done. One physiologist has said that sustained mental work is out of the question at anything over 10,000 feet. We certainly could not agree with this. Those who have read Norton's despatches to the *Times*, especially one dictated at Camp III, when he was burdened with anxiety and partially blind, will admit that this effort from 21,000 feet was not a bad intellectual performance. The main effect of altitude is a mental laziness which determination can overcome.

I made some mental tests on the members of the party. These tests were very simple. The first was a multiplication test. It consisted in multiplying the figures 123456789 by 7. The second was a division test, and consisted in dividing the same series of figures by 9. A record was made at successive altitudes of the time taken to do these sums. Probably these tests were far too simple. By an effort of concentration they could be easily done, and thus the effect of altitude was not properly shown. I give the results for what they are worth. They show no definite deterioration of mental activity. It will not please the members of the next expedition to hear that more complicated and worrying tests are required.

Multiplication test, showing time in seconds for completion of sum

Altitude in feet	R.W.H.	B.B.	E.F.N.	G.L.M.	T.H.S.	E.O.S.	G.B.	J.V.H.	A.C.I.	N.E.O.
0	20	—	—	—	—	—	—	—	—	—
7000	25	25	27	13	40	43	40	35	25	80
14,300	25	24	19	15	28	43	25	—	28	—
16,500	18	23	28	17	40	35	35	55	35	30
21,000	17	—	—	—	—	35	27	40	—	—

Division test, showing time in seconds for completion of sum

Altitude in feet	R.W.H.	B.B.	E.F.N.	G.L.M.	T.H.S.	E.O.S.	G.B.	J.V.H.	A.C.I.	N.E.O.
0	30	—	—	—	—	—	—	—	—	—
7000	20	20	30	10	25	55	15	35	15	45
14,300	28	20	13	23	20	45	17	—	17	—
16,500	13	27	23	17	40	38	23	43	20	50
21,000	15	—	—	—	—	40	13	59	—	—

The knee-jerks were examined at successive altitudes. In no case did they seem in any way affected by the height. Three of the party developed mild tremors: one a tremor of the eyelids at 14,000 feet, two a fine tremor of the fingers at 21,000 feet. This was an indication of nervous strain.

It was a common sign of exhaustion and anxiety amongst those serving in the great war.

SLEEP

To my mind insomnia was an unpleasant feature. But there were others who suffered from no lack of sleep except when they happened to be cold. Bruce on two nights slept for more than ten hours at 21,000 feet. He had a fair, but somewhat broken, night at 23,000 feet. He had about two hours' sleep at the beginning of the night, then a long period of sleeplessness, then a few more hours' sleep in the morning, when at 25,000 feet. He always slept with his head raised, having learned the trick on the previous expedition. Somervell slept well at 25,000 feet, and had two good spells of sleep at 27,000 feet. Norton, however, takes the record. He slept well and had an excellent night at 27,000 feet. A point about high altitude sleeplessness is the fact that it is not associated with restlessness, nor does it cause weariness the next day. One lies awake, but does not toss about; nor is the sleep accompanied with irritable dreams.

GLACIER LASSITUDE

A distinct feature in the Mount Everest region is the very pronounced glacier lassitude which develops over tracts of ice. This was most marked on the Rongbuk glacier, especially when passing through a trough in the ice at an altitude of about 20,000 feet. The trough was a remarkable feature, being girt on either side with walls of ice in many places hewn into fantastic pinnacles and ornamented with pyramidal spires. In this trough there was a peculiar sapping of energy, a weakness of the legs, and a disinclination to move. It was not a breathlessness due to exertion, but a loss of muscular power. There was a feeling of prostration. One seemed to drag oneself along, instead of going with the usual strength. A profuse sweating was not uncommon. It was something like the oppression experienced when marching through a hot moist jungle in the rains. The lassitude appeared immediately after stepping on to the glacier; it was as quickly relieved on again reaching rock or moraine. It was most noticeable in the absence of wind and in the middle of the day when the sun was strong. It was absent late at evening and in the early morning, and was less marked on cloudy days.

The cause of this lassitude is easily explained. The conditions for its development are a sheet of ice, a hot sun, and a still air. The sun melts the superficial layer of the ice. The lowest stratum of the atmosphere becomes saturated with moisture but does not rise owing to its being chilled by contact with the ice. Thus, when on the glacier, one is in a saturated atmosphere, and this, in conjunction with the high altitude, is sufficient to cause the unpleasant effects.

We did not notice that other atmospheric conditions had any special influence on these high altitude symptoms. This was different from my experiences in the western Himalaya. There, on two occasions, our party climbed the same peak to a height of 18,203 feet. During the first ascent the sky was clear, the air was free from moisture, and our disability was slight. On the second occasion the conditions were different. The sky was dark, stormy weather was imminent, and the atmosphere felt heavy and damp. Our distress on this second occasion was acute. Every few paces found us gasping for breath, and we had repeatedly to make short halts. The same explanation applies to this as in the case of the glacier lassitude. On the second ascent the atmosphere was laden with moisture. The free evaporation of perspiration was checked, and, as a consequence, the high altitude symptoms were increased.

Individual Variation

The experiences of the party, as already detailed, indicate considerable individual variation with respect to oxygen want. It was obvious that some of us breathed more laboriously than others. One suffered from headache, another did not; one lost the sense of taste, another observed no such change; one was sleepless at comparatively low altitudes, another slept well at the highest camps. One member seemed particularly resistant to the lassitude that occurs over snow and ice. All were agreed that the Sherpa porters suffered, on an average, less than Europeans. Their power of carrying loads was extraordinary. They went with loads as fast as did the climbers without loads. It was not that they were muscularly more powerful than we. Probably their actual strength was less. It was their capacity to carry that was so much greater. This must be due to their permanent habitations being at altitudes of 12,000 to 14,000 feet, and to the fact that they habitually carry loads over passes of 16,000 and 18,000 feet.

Oxygen

To what extent does the breathing of oxygen alleviate the symptoms already described? Theoretically we should expect an enormous benefit. We know of its great value in balloon ascents, which could not be made to extreme altitudes unless oxygen was breathed. But our evidence on the subject is most unsatisfactory. The two climbers who could have told us most about it have perished on the mountain. Bruce used oxygen on his ascent to the North Col—that is, between 21,000 and 23,000 feet. He noticed scarcely any benefit. Odell used it at the same altitude and considered that it gave no relief. Later he used it between 25,000 and 27,000 feet. There the oxygen seemed to relieve the breathing and diminish the tiredness of the legs. He thinks it may have helped to keep up the temperature. Its use produced an uncomfortable drying of the throat which necessitated frequent swallowing and expectoration. He abandoned the oxygen at 27,000 feet and descended easily without it. It is remarkable how little benefit was obtained from the oxygen compared with the experiences of the previous expedition.

Acclimatisation

I pass to the problem of acclimatisation. When we compare a rapid with a gradual ascent we see how powerful is this factor of adaptation to increasing heights. Haldane describes the condition of visitors after a rapid ascent of Pike's Peak to a height of only 14,100 feet. "Many persons walked or rode up during the night to see the sun rise, especially on Sunday morning, and the scene in the restaurant and on the platform outside can only be likened to that on the deck or in the cabin of a cross-channel steamer during rough weather." Now the altitude at which this scene took place was about the same as that of the Tibetan plateau. But our ascent to the plateau was gradual, and therefore accompanied by acclimatisation. As a consequence we felt scarcely any distress. We were quite comfortable at a height where, if our ascent had been rapidly made, we should have been like the nauseated visitors on Pike's Peak.

But the contrast is more marked if we compare our progress with an air ascent. In the year 1875 Tissandier and his two companions made their famous ascent in a balloon from Paris. They were provided with oxygen but were unable to make use of it. Tissandier fainted at 26,500 feet, and when he recovered consciousness the balloon was descending and his companions were dead. The balloon had reached an altitude of 27,950 feet. This was a rapid ascent with no acclimatisation. The result was death between 26,000 and 28,000 feet even when sitting quietly in a balloon. Compare this with a gradual attack on Mount Everest. Climbers without oxygen have ascended the mountain to 28,000 feet, somewhere about the same height where death occurred in the balloon. Yet at that altitude they were capable of strenuous effort; they showed no indication of fainting; they could sleep well at a slightly lower elevation, and were comparatively comfortable so long as they were at rest. The difference in the two ascents is due to acclimatisation, without which any attempt to reach the summit of Mount Everest would be altogether out of the question. The fact is that balloon ascents and experiments in air-chambers are not at all comparable to the conditions of a prolonged climb.

A special point which the expedition of this year taught us is that persons who have once experienced high altitudes will acclimatise very much more rapidly than those entering them for the first time. Those of our party who had been on two expeditions were unanimous in the view that they suffered less on the second than on the first occasion. One said that his mind was much more active than it was in 1922, another that he reached Camp III with much less difficulty, another that he had not to breathe deeply at night as he had found necessary on the previous expedition. Also it was obvious that the new members of the party were distinctly more affected than the old. This is a point of practical importance. It means that, other things being equal, old hands will acclimatise more rapidly and be in a fitter state to climb the mountain than will be a party of fresh recruits. Even aviators have noticed the same thing. Although their ascents are so quick and short, yet they say that they get accustomed to the height. The body seems, as it were, to become trained by one experience, and therefore to make the necessary adjustments more easily on reaching high altitudes a second time.

To what height can acclimatisation continue? There seems to be no doubt of a steady improvement at 19,000 feet. Shebbeare spent over a month at that altitude in Camp II. At first he found the ascent to Camp III very laborious, but at the end of a month could do it with ease, and on the last day did it in the record time of 1 hour 55 minutes. Odell remained for ten days at 23,000 feet, and said that he certainly felt better as a result of this. Somervell believed that acclimatisation took place at 24,000 feet. But we must remember that while acclimatisation is in progress there may be physical deterioration at the same time. Though the body is becoming more accustomed to the altitude, yet simultaneously it is losing both in weight and strength. Dr Kellas puts the important question: "Is it possible to become sufficiently acclimatised to altitudes of 24,000 feet to 26,000 feet to enable one to climb to over 29,000 feet?" I think that most of our party would reply in the affirmative. Two of them have already reached 28,000 feet aided by no other power beyond their own natural capacities for acclimatisation.

AFTER-EFFECTS

A note as to the after-effects consequent on residence at the high camps. The climbers were examined before we left the mountain. All of them showed signs of dilatation of the heart; in two it was decidedly marked. All were debilitated. All had wasted considerably—probably as much as 1½ to 2 stone. The porters too had lost much weight. Barcroft observed the same effect on his expedition to Peru. Loss of weight occurred in all the members of his party, the most marked being a decline from 155 to 131 lbs. in twenty-seven days.

Those of the expedition who had been badly frostbitten required treatment for weeks after we had left the mountain. Frostbite showed itself in two varieties: the moist form with large blisters full of fluid and the dry gangrenous type. Snow-blindness also may need after-treatment. A point of interest was that Norton developed a severe attack of blindness when at high altitudes though in the absence of snow. At 28,000 feet he was on bare rock. He thought it unnecessary to use his snow-glasses, and on the next day he was completely blind. The sun's rays in this thin air can cause a most acute attack of conjunctivitis even when reflected from bare dark rock.

Thus life on the mountain causes physical deterioration. Improvement followed on our return to the base camp, with increase in appetite and better sleep. Finally we descended into the Rongshar valley, where, at the pleasant altitude of 10,000 feet, all were quickly restored to health.

CONCLUSION

A last word on the possibility of reaching the summit. In the year 1916, at an afternoon meeting of this society, Dr Kellas showed an interesting dissociation curve of oxy-haemoglobin in blood. On this curve he plotted the heights of some well-known mountains. From it he drew the following deductions. "The curve," he said, "is very suggestive. It shows that the strain on the climber is nearly negligible up to 10,000 feet, and at about 15,000 feet becomes appreciable; but one must pass above 20,000 feet before the steepening of the curve indicates that the mountaineer will have to adapt himself carefully to his aerial environment. At 23,000 feet the curve is getting much steeper, and the climber will obviously be put on his mettle above 25,000 feet, for the curve then attains its steepest. Every 1000 feet still higher must mean considerably increased difficulty, and the climber near the summit of Mount Everest will probably be on his last reserves in the way of acclimatisation and strength." This deduction was made before the first assault on Everest, and I think that we can now safely say that our practical experiences bear it out.

I think that climbers will reach the summit of Mount Everest even without the help of oxygen. Though the physiological difficulties are undoubtedly severe, yet they can be overcome. But the condition of the weather must be more favourable than this year. The climbers must be in perfect health and in first-rate training; they must be men of exceptional powers of endurance, and their capacity for acclimatisation must be complete.

APPENDIX II

THE nature of acclimatisation had, unknown to me, been the subject of systematic thought by Cecil Murray during 1924, i.e., at the time when I was writing the concluding chapter of the present volume. The beautiful quantitative way in which Murray has expressed himself makes my own statement appear very crude; I have asked him to let me publish his chart showing the correlation of the principal factors in the respiratory system. Any of my readers may, from the data given in this book or elsewhere, fill in the chart for a particular person under given circumstances. Among other things he will see whether the data hang together or are incompatible. The following is Murray's description:

Fig. 52 was designed to illustrate graphically the Distribution of Function among the factors involved in the supply of oxygen to the body. There are four quadrants, each representing a simple relationship according to the following equations:

$$\Delta p' \times DC = MR \qquad\qquad \dots\dots(1),$$

$$\Delta O_2 \% \times SHF = 10\Delta p' \qquad\qquad \dots\dots(2),$$

$$\Delta O_2 \% \times Hgb = 10{,}000\Delta O_2 \text{ c.c.} \qquad\qquad \dots\dots(3),$$

$$1000\Delta O_2 \text{ c.c.} \times BF = MR \qquad\qquad \dots\dots(4).$$

$\Delta p'$ is the "mean" head of oxygen pressure, in mm. of mercury, existing between alveolar air and blood of a composition varying, along the length of a capillary, from venous to arterial (or, the mean head of pressure between blood varying from arterial to venous composition and the average oxygen pressure of the tissues).

DC is a measure of the diffusing capacity of the capillary bed—it may be thought of as being proportional to the active capillary surface area.

MR is the oxygen consumption, in c.c. oxygen (standard) per minute of the individual—the metabolic rate. Equation (1) is a simple application of the law of diffusion, and serves also to define the unit of DC.

$\Delta O_2 \%$ is the coefficient of utilisation—the difference in per cent. saturation between arterial and mixed-venous bloods (taking 100 % saturation to include the dissolved free oxygen).

SHF is the specific haemoglobin flow—the ratio of the product $Hgb \times BF$ to DC. The term emphasises the physiological adjustment of the haemoglobin flow, HF, to the capillary area. The reciprocal relationship has been called the specific diffusing capacity, SDC. Thus

$$SHF = \frac{1}{SDC} = \frac{Hgb \times BF}{DC} = \frac{HF}{DC}.$$

Hgb is the total oxygen capacity of the blood in volumes per cent.

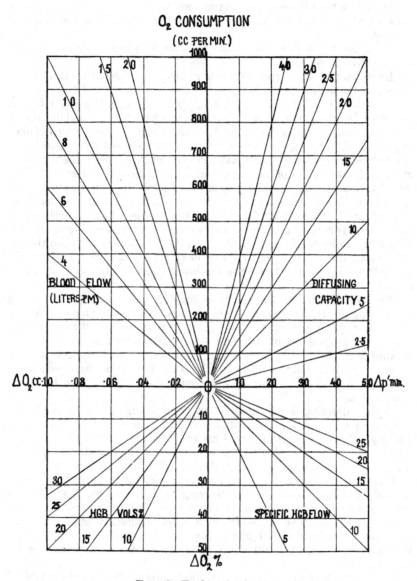

Fig. 52. Explanation in text.

ΔO_2 c.c. is the difference in oxygen content, in c.c. O_2 per c.c. of blood, between arterial and venous bloods. Equation (3) expresses an obvious relation.

BF is the blood flow per minute, measured in litres. Equation (4) is also an obvious relation.

Equation (2) will be seen to follow directly from the other three equations and the definition of SHF.

In so far as diffusion operates in oxygen exchange, the above factors describe the process with considerable completeness. It will be noted, however, that the term $\Delta p'$ is not one which can be directly determined experimentally. It can be derived from an independent determination of the diffusing capacity or the diffusion coefficient, taken with the metabolic rate. If, however, the properties of blood are known, the arterial and the mixed-venous points, and the pO_2 of alveolar air (or of tissues); $\Delta p'$ can be evaluated by means of a graphical integration. The relationship between $\Delta p'$ and ΔO_2 % for all possible combinations of arterial and venous bloods at varying hydrogen ion activities and varying oxygen pressures in alveolar air and in tissues has been worked out on the basis of the diffusion theory. This data will be presented in the form of twenty-one charts with a coordinate background exactly like the lower right quadrant of the figure shown.

Now on this figure the conditions for diffusion of oxygen prevailing in the lung are represented by a rectangle, a corner of which lies in each of the four quadrants of the figure. Another rectangle, differing only in respect to the position of the right side, would represent the conditions prevailing in the tissues (other than the lung) as a whole. For a more complete treatment of what may be said to constitute the physico-chemical background of the diffusion process, reference should be made to the papers cited (1), (2), (3).

Such a description of the physical background is not superfluous. Only by pushing a theory to its logical limit is it possible to test its validity. Moreover, certain problems are perhaps brought into clearer relief. The rectangle alluded to exhibits by its specific shape the distribution of function among the coordinated components. What re-distribution takes place when factors in the environment or in the individual become altered? In studying such questions, what factors will the experimenter choose to determine? What physiological laws delimit a certain range upon the wide physico-chemical scheme? What laws determine the actual correlation between variables which from the purely physico-chemical point of view are to all appearances independent?

Such considerations have led Professor Barcroft into that field of Physiology which is most perfectly adapted to the study of the problem of Adaptation. The peculiar fitness of the subject of oxygen exchange lies in the simple physiological requirement for this gas, the complex components their inter-relations satisfy this need, and the relative ease with which by which the whole subject can be approached and probed in a quantitative manner. In this last sense especially, the respiratory function, among all physiological functions, is absolutely unique.

REFERENCES

(1) HENDERSON, L. J., BOCK, A. V., FIELD, H. jr. AND STODDARD, J. L. *Journal of Biological Chemistry*, LIX. 379. 1924.

(2) HENDERSON, L. J. AND MURRAY, C. D.

(3) MURRAY, C. D. AND MORGAN, W. O. P. (These last two will be submitted in the near future to the *Journal of Biological Chemistry*.)

BARCROFT, BOYCOTT, DUNN and PETERS[1] have measured, among other things, the following variables in normal goats: (1) MR, (2) r.p.m. (respirations per minute), (3) and (4) pO_2 and pCO_2 (of *expired* air, in mm. Hg), (5) and (6) $A \%$ and $V \%$ (per cent. saturations of arterial and mixed-venous bloods from the heart), (7) $\Delta O_2 \%$, (8) BF, (9) ΔO_2 c.c., and (10) Hgb. The notation and units, unless otherwise stated, are the same as in Appendix II. Such data are fairly well suited for a study illustrative of physiological organisation—the problem suggested by the questions raised in Appendix II and throughout the book. From two to five experiments were performed on ten goats, with a total of thirty experiments. The data have been used to determine the correlation coefficients between each pair of the ten factors selected. For this purpose, for each variable, deviations, from the mean value in the *respective individual goat*, were tabulated. Thus the deviations may be treated as if they occurred in a hypothetical, average, individual goat, and the result is a picture of average individual physiology. (If deviations in any one factor had been taken from a single mean value obtained by averaging for the ten goats, the result would perhaps be equally interesting, but its significance would be quite different. This would be comparative physiology *among* individuals.) The correlation coefficients (r), calculated from the data mentioned, are given in Table I. It will be remembered that the coefficient can, in general, assume any value from $+1$ to -1.

Table I. *Partial correlation coefficients. Zero order*

	1	2	3	4	5	6	7	8	9	10
	MR	r.p.m.	pO_2	pCO_2	$A \%$	$V \%$	$\Delta O_2 \%$	BF	ΔO_2 c.c.	Hgb
σ	12·5	1·61	2·05	1·85	4·01	4·66	4·92	·338	·0057	·453
MR	—	+·336	−·013	+·213	−·186	−·300	+·065	+·395	+·358	+·420
r.p.m.	—	—	−·013	−·006	+·186	−·170	+·316	−·034	+·288	+·088
pO_2	—	—	—	−·379	+·212	+·010	+·009	−·160	+·103	·000
pCO_2	—	—	—	—	−·336	−·380	+·010	−·028	+·248	+·358
$A \%$	—	—	—	—	—	+·396	+·443	−·433	+·328	−·084
$V \%$	—	—	—	—	—	—	−·660	+·359	−·471	+·031
$\Delta O_2 \%$	—	—	—	—	—	—	—	−·706	+·765	−·069
BF	—	—	—	—	—	—	—	—	−·700	+·012
ΔO_2 c.c.	—	—	—	—	—	—	—	—	—	+·398

In the table, by way of example, the correlation between metabolic rate and respiration rate, r_{12}, is $+·336$. This is a measure of the regularity with which high values of MR and high values for r.p.m. are, in this case positively, associated—and similarly for low values. The proportionality constants (for the two regression equations) are obtained by the following equations:

$$MR = r_{12} \frac{\sigma_{MR}}{\sigma_{\text{r.p.m.}}} \times \text{r.p.m.} = K_{12}\,\text{r.p.m.},$$

and

$$\text{r.p.m.} = r_{12} \frac{\sigma_{\text{r.p.m.}}}{\sigma_{MR}} \times MR = K_{21}\,MR.$$

Here σ_{MR} and $\sigma_{\text{r.p.m.}}$ are the standard deviations of MR and r.p.m. in the respective proper units. The first equation yields the "best value" for MR, in the range studied, if it was to be calculated from r.p.m. Moreover, the constant, K_{12}, shows by how much the metabolic rate has increased for a given increase in the rate of respiration. The second equation gives "best values" for r.p.m. in terms of MR.

At first sight it might be expected that the correlation between MR and r.p.m. would be much higher, perhaps ·8 or more. It would, undoubtedly in an experiment lasting a short time, in a single individual, granting a high degree of experimental accuracy, if the range of metabolism were small. But from day to day, as circumstances vary, an individual may vary in his response, so that at one time the response is an increased *depth* of breathing. In constructing an average individual such variations will be all the more effective in lowering the coefficient. With this in mind, the number + ·336, for the "average individual," may be considered as relatively high and as indicating a fairly universal correlation and proportionality constants of roughly similar order in the responses of various individuals.

From the above table further sets of coefficients may be calculated, excluding one factor after another, in the attempt to keep the conditions constant and thus study the "true" relation between any two factors. For instance, the correlation between r.p.m. and BF, r_{28}, is − ·034. What would the correlation become if the metabolic rate were kept constant? To find r_{28} the following equation is used

$$r_{28} = \frac{r_{28} - r_{21} \cdot r_{81}}{(1 - r_{21}{}^2)^{\frac{1}{2}} (1 - r_{81}{}^2)^{\frac{1}{2}}} = -\,·193.$$

The result is an indication, among other things, that increase in respiration rate relieves the blood flow, that is, the heart—and *vice versa*. Since r.p.m. and BF are both positively associated with MR, it is obvious that the tendency toward a negative or inverse correlation between r.p.m. and BF (which really exists under all conditions) is less clearly discernible when the metabolic rate is allowed to vary, and is made much clearer if this "disturbing factor" is kept constant. Essentially the process of calculation is a device by which corrections can be made for variations in MR.

Table II gives the coefficients between other pairs of factors *at constant metabolic rate*. Nine other similar tables, keeping each factor in turn constant, could be made, then every *pair* of factors could be kept constant, every set of three factors, etc., etc.!

Table II. *Partial correlation coefficients. First order. MR constant*

	3 pO_2	4 pCO_2	5 A %	6 V %	7 ΔO_2 %	8 BF	9 ΔO_2 c.c.	10 Hgb
r.p.m.	– ·007	– ·072	+ ·268	– ·078	+ ·313	– ·193	+ ·191	– ·062
pO_2	—	– ·385	+ ·217	+ ·006	+ ·010	– ·169	+ ·116	+ ·006
pCO_2	—	—	– ·308	– ·339	– ·004	– ·125	+ ·189	+ ·304
A %	—	—	—	+ ·363	+ ·464	– ·399	+ ·431	– ·007
V %	—	—	—	—	– ·674	+ ·545	– ·408	+ ·181
ΔO_2 %	—	—	—	—	—	– ·800	+ ·792	– ·106
BF	—	—	—	—	—	—	– ·982	– ·187
ΔO_2 c.c.	—	—	—	—	—	—	—	+ ·293

Many of the correlations are obvious, some perhaps are unreliable, due to errors in calculation which are very difficult to avoid, some are evidently high because they involve variables which are arithmetically derived and hence not subject to experimental error, but others are undoubtedly suggestive. It seems, to take a single instance only, that the high correlation between MR and Hgb, $+ ·420$, is of special interest in view of Professor Barcroft's recent work on the spleen as a mobile store of haemoglobin.

There is a general, though partly negative, conclusion, suggested by a consideration of Table I, which is forced upon us. There is no *unique* respiratory stimulus. An attempt to define the exact meaning of the term is sufficient to indicate the difficulty involved in the concept. There may be a hundred mechanisms, the operation of any one of which, all other independent factors being kept constant, may be followed directly and invariably by increased respiration. But physiologically, respiration and all similar types of function, are only partly correlated with the factors or mechanisms which have or have not been the object of special researches. The high values of the correlation between r.p.m. and ΔO_2 % indicates that respiration is more highly correlated with the coefficient of utilisation than with any of the other factors included in this discussion. The stimulus of any function must be sought in the complex organisation of many factors contributing in varying degrees to the resulting effect.

REFERENCE

(1) Barcroft, J., Boycott, A. E., Dunn, J. S. and Peters, R. A. *Quart. Journ. of Med.* xiii. 35. 1919.

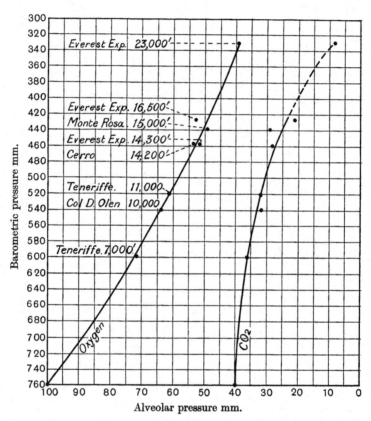

FIG. 53. Correlation of altitude with alveolar pressures of oxygen and carbonic acid.
The Everest results are taken from Dr Somervell's paper, *Journal of Physiology*,
LX, p. 282, 1925. Each point is the average of a number of determinations.

INDEX

Printed in the United States
By Bookmasters